THE
WHITLOCK
WORKOUT

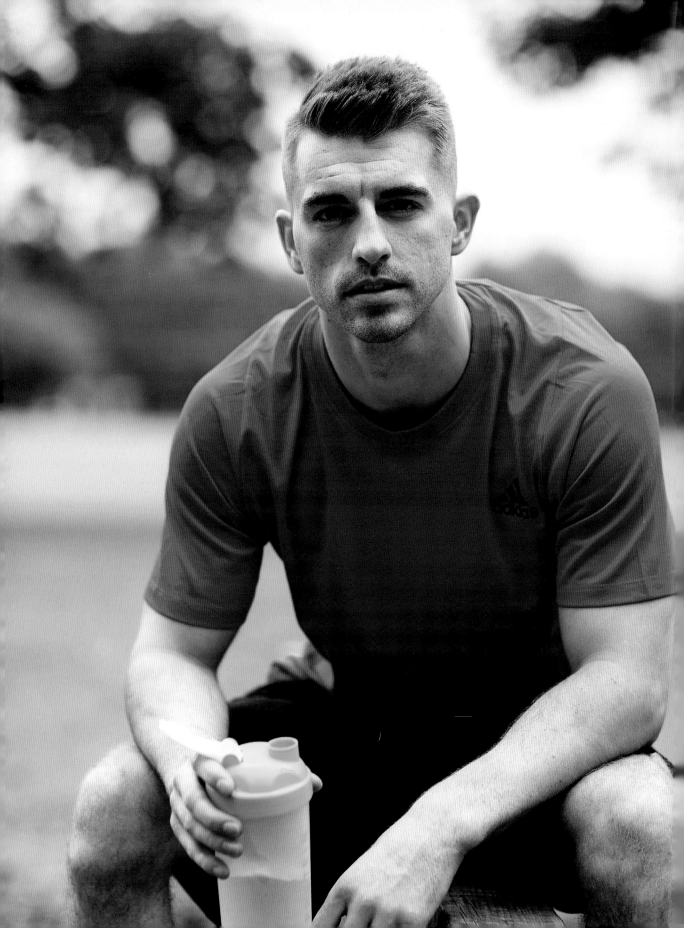

THE
WHITLOCK
WORKOUT

GET FIT AND HEALTHY IN MINUTES
WITH MAX WHITLOCK

PHOTOGRAPHY BY DAN JONES

I want to dedicate this book to everyone who has followed my journey,
my family who have been amazing support throughout and to
everyone who wants to achieve their health and fitness goals.

I wish you all the best!

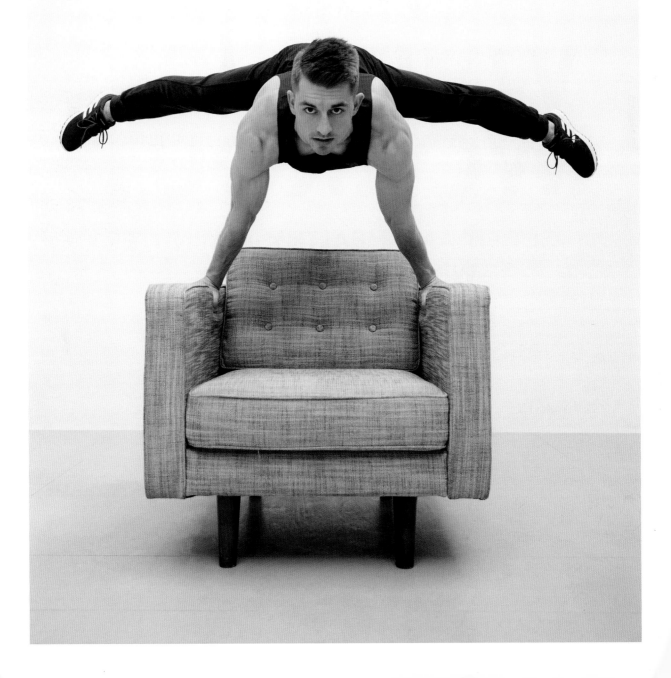

CONTENTS

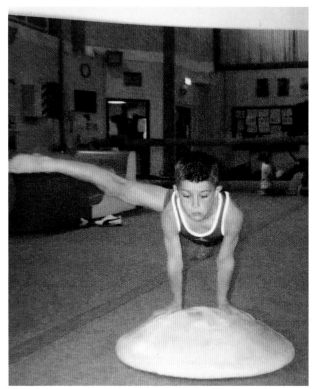

Working on the 'mushroom', which is a piece of training equipment for the pommel horse, when I was nine.

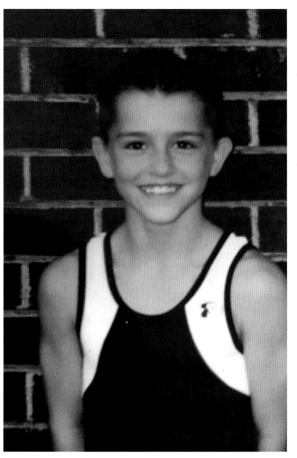

Ten years old and proudly wearing my regional team kit.

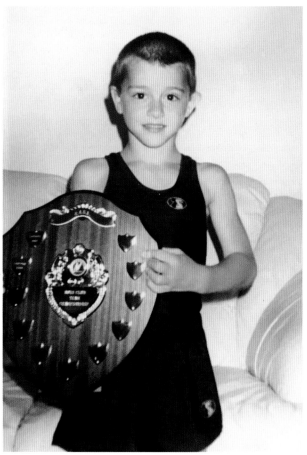

Holding a shield we won for a team competition when I was eight. It was my first competition!

INTRODUCTION

MY LIFE SO FAR

When I get the chance to sit down and take a breath, I realise just how crazy my life has turned out. Olympic golds, world titles, an MBE, getting married to my amazing wife Leah, the birth of my beautiful daughter Willow – and writing this book! Looking back, I can see that it all stems from having been lucky enough to have found a sport I love and putting a lot of hard work and dedication into it.

EARLY YEARS

I was born in Hemel Hempstead in 1993 and I enjoyed all sports when I was young but I gravitated towards swimming, following in the wake of my brother, and was a member of my local club. I still really enjoy being in the water when I go on holidays but it's definitely more about leisurely floating and splashing about in the sun rather than ploughing out lengths these days. At the age of seven, though, a mate of mine at the swimming club, who was also doing gymnastics, persuaded me and my older brother to come and have a go. I fell in love with it immediately. I seemed to have a build that suited it and, two years later at the age of nine, I was selected for the GB squad. At that time, with my hours in the gym ramping up, I had to make a decision to commit to either gymnastics or swimming. It wasn't a hard choice as gymnastics was going so well and I was really enjoying it, but I did miss the pool and my mates at the club.

Along with having to make that choice between swimming and gymnastics, I also needed to fit in school somewhere. It was tricky sometimes, especially as I got older and the amount of both my homework and training started ramping up. I made the decision to study BTEC Sport, which taught me the importance of time management and I learned some valuable lessons about gym/life balance. I've also been incredibly lucky in having a really supportive family.

My parents have been amazing. I hate to think of the amount of miles they've driven taking me to training and competitions, but their support has been so much more than just ferrying me about. They have always struck the perfect balance between being supportive but never pushy. I always felt sure that, if I stopped enjoying my gymnastics and wanted to try something else, they would have supported my decision 100 per cent. Knowing this made a massive difference; it seemed to take some of the pressure off when I was competing because it was more about enjoyment than winning. I think this has played a huge part in my developing a fairly relaxed and chilled attitude to competition, which I feel has contributed greatly to my success. My parents have also been brilliant in managing my expectations throughout my career. I'm sure that coaches told them that I had talent but they never passed this on to me and just let me have fun. This has really helped to shape my mindset and I always try to just focus on enjoying the process, not fixating on expectations, letting the results take care of themselves.

SLOVENIAN ADVENTURE

When I was twelve, I had to make a massive decision. My coach Klemen Bedenik was planning to return home to Slovenia and he wanted me to go with him and train at the gym he was going to be coaching at. I remember sitting down with my parents and talking it through. I was really young, very shy and lacking in confidence and so it was a scary prospect. They were so supportive, though, didn't push me at all and I came to the decision that I had to give it a go or I might regret it for ever.

I flew out on my own, lived with Klemen and his family and, although I was only there for three months, it felt like a lifetime. I got really homesick, would call home every day and, although I definitely learned a lot, it eventually all got too much and I decided to come home. I didn't have any regrets about going to Slovenia or coming back; it was something I had to try and, again, I'm immensely grateful to my parents for giving me the space to make those decisions. While I was out in Slovenia, I met my current coach, Scott Hann. He was there with a group of boys from South Essex Gymnastics Club on a training camp and I got to know them all quite well. When I returned home, I got in touch with Scott straight away, asked if I could join and he told me to come in the very next day. South Essex has been my club ever since.

DELHI 2010 COMMONWEALTH GAMES

The 2010 Commonwealth Games in Delhi was my first big international competition and, at just seventeen, going to India and taking part in a massive multi-country and multi-sport event was pretty overwhelming. It fell really close to the World Championships where all the top British gymnasts were competing, and this gave me and some other juniors a chance at the Commonwealths. It was a huge opportunity. Although I came back with two silvers and a bronze, which I was delighted with, I knew I'd made mistakes that had cost me better medals, and that certainly fired me up. Looking back, it was the first time that I thought I might be able to really achieve something in the sport. I was never one of those kids who always dreamed of going to the Olympics, as I just enjoyed my gymnastics and took things one step at a time. Even after the Commonwealths, I was only really thinking about my next step up in terms of competition, maybe going to the senior European Champs but not much beyond that. I think this attitude helped me stay grounded, to keep enjoying the sport. For me it's still my fun 'hobby'.

LONDON 2012

Going into 2011, though, I couldn't ignore the growing sense of expectation in the country of a home Olympics and obviously I wanted to be on the team. The 2011 World Champs were in Tokyo and I was in a real scrap for a place on the team. I flew out and it was only with four days to go before competition that I got the devastating news that I hadn't made the team and had been picked as a reserve. It was a real blow at the time but actually it turned into a bit of a blessing in disguise as it pushed me to work even harder in the gym. I got my chance at the London 2012 demonstration event at the O2 – the team's final chance to qualify. We had a brilliant event, and the whole team qualified but I still wasn't a certainty for the Olympics. I had to prove myself in competition, and so I embarked on a gruelling and really stressful year. It seemed like one competition after another and they didn't all go well. I fell off, three competitions in a row, but eventually – and just in time – it all came right and I made the team. It had been a real fight, both with my own doubts and with my rivals, and I'd pushed myself harder than ever before, but I learned so much in terms of determination and resilience.

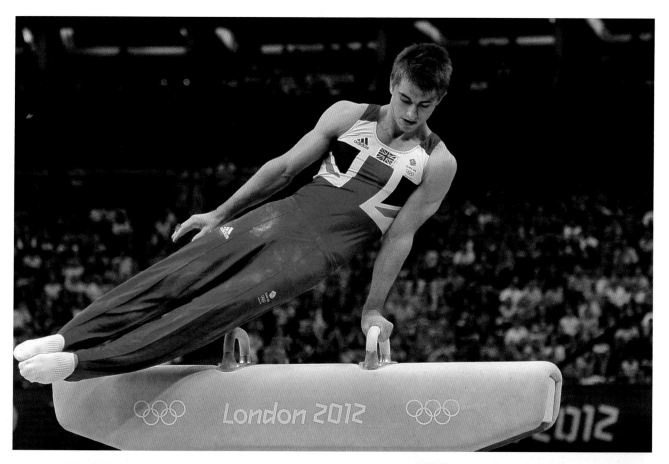

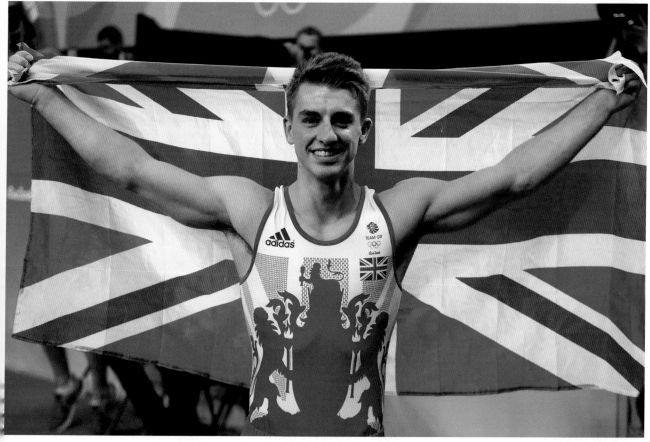

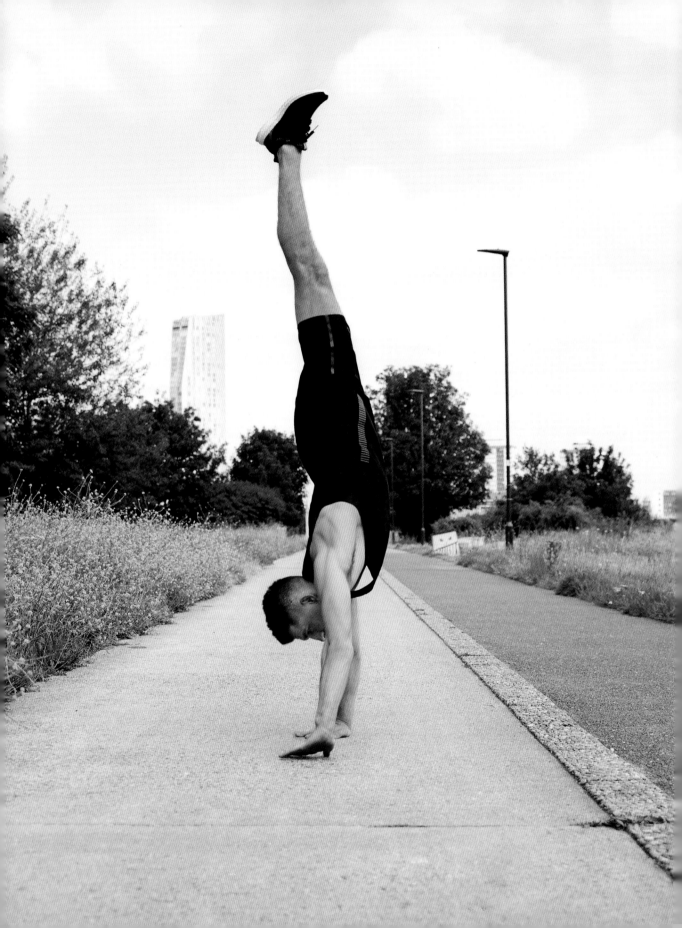

The actual lead-up to the Games was a bit weird because we were in a real bubble and missed out on all the hype. In the Olympic Village you got a sense that the nation was coming together and really getting behind Team GB but we were so focused before our events that we had no idea quite how great the excitement was. It was only when I stepped out into the competition arena that it really hit me. It was during the team final and we'd put ourselves in a position where we might be able to scrape a medal. I never like to know what the previous gymnasts have scored or the position I'm in, but the roar of the crowd left me with no doubt. I was so young, had never even competed in a senior World Champs but here I was in a medal scrap at a home Olympics. The rest of the guys and I held it together, nailed our routines and we won the first team medal in gymnastics for over 100 years!

With an Olympic medal in the bank, it really took the pressure off, and when I made the final of the pommel horse, I was able to just enjoy it. When I was walking out for my routine, the score of the guy before me popped up on the screen and I couldn't avoid seeing it. It was a huge score and all I could do was laugh and think that I might as well just go for it. I managed the best routine I'd ever performed up to that point in my career and, unbelievably, managed to win another bronze medal. Looking back, London 2012 stands out so much for me because it was such a battle just getting there and then the actual Games were like a fairytale.

BETWEEN THE GAMES

In hindsight it was almost inevitable that there was going to be a bit of a comedown after the incredible high of 2012, but it was a tough few years. 2013 and 2014 went well, with more international medals, but then I had a really bad competition at the Worlds in 2014. Gymnastics is so tough in this regard because you've got to hit every move perfectly on the day. You might have nailed a routine loads of times in training but all it takes is one small mistake on a competition day, which is obviously frustrating for any athlete, yet that is what competition is all about.

I think, though, that I've learned more from the competitions that haven't gone quite to plan and, once you accept that you can't be perfect all of the time and that mistakes are normal, it makes you a far more robust competitor. No matter how badly an event goes, I find that I'm always able to take some positives from it and know that I'll get another chance. This isn't just mindless optimism; having this sort of mindset has been crucial to me having a long career for a gymnast and not burning out.

Going into 2015 I really felt as though the bad results were behind me, especially after a fantastic Commonwealth Games in Glasgow, and that I was hitting peak fitness and form at the perfect time in the build-up to Rio. I remember coming home from training one day absolutely buzzing and telling Mum and Dad how strong I felt and that I was performing all of my routines better and more consistently than ever. Literally within a week, it all fell apart and I barely had the stamina to get through a single routine. Then, when I was working on the parallel bars, I got completely disoriented in the air and landed badly on my head. Scott said enough was enough, that it was getting dangerous and, rather than trying to push on and keep getting frustrated, we took our foot off the gas. I went for blood tests and it turned out I had glandular fever. It wasn't great timing being so close to Rio but getting the diagnosis was a real relief. I now knew why my fitness had slumped and, although there was nothing I could do but rest, at least it was an explicable rut that I should be able to get out of.

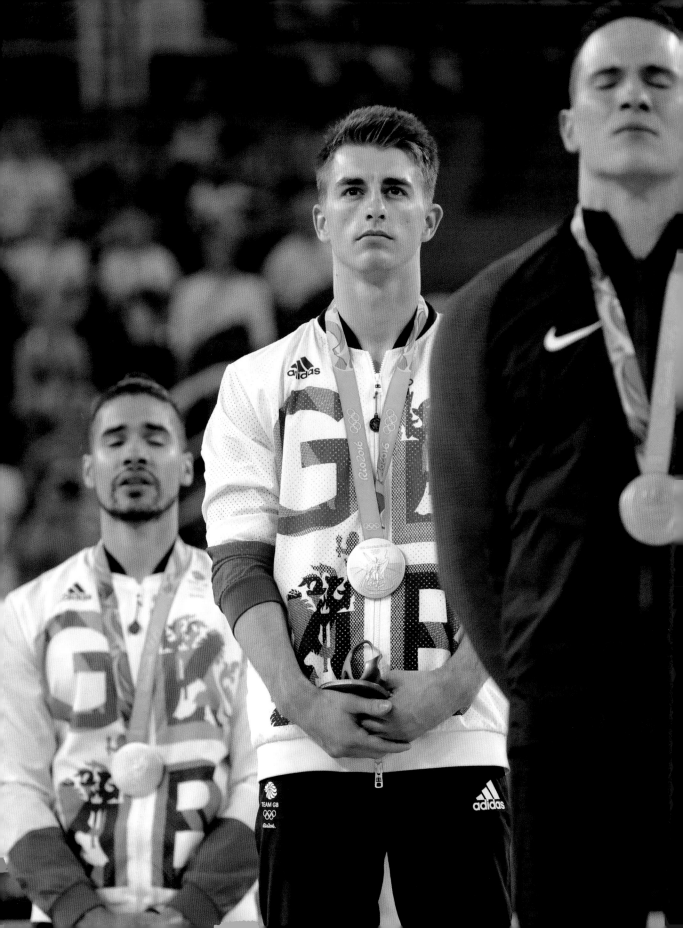

Resting up was all well and good in theory but there's always a battle between your rational brain and your competitive brain and they don't always agree. The European Champs were looming and I really wanted to take part. To qualify I had to take part in the British Champs, which I limped through with a substandard routine and very little training and just about managed to get a spot on the team. I was running on fumes and, because my preparation and fitness were woefully inadequate, I made a load of mistakes and really shouldn't have been there. All it did was prolong the illness but it finally got the message through to me that I had to take some time out.

I went on holiday and, as well as giving me the time I needed to recover physically, it also gave me an invaluable opportunity to assess how I trained and competed. I'd seen so many gymnasts burn out by trying to train the same way later on in their career as when they were fresh juniors and I had been doing the same. If I wanted to get well, back to full fitness and have a long career, I had to start training smarter and avoid overtraining. I had to accept that my body could no longer cope with the huge volume of training that I used to do and I had to make the time I spent in the gym far more efficient. The emphasis really had to switch to quality rather than quantity and I had to start making my recovery as much of a priority.

Sometimes you just get days when you feel sluggish, your arms and body feel heavy and everything is a struggle. In the past, on those days, I probably would have pushed on through, trained just for the sake of logging the hours and simply gone through the motions. The problem with that, though, is, when you're training in the gym, if you're not feeling strong and focused, you're not going to be safe and are more likely to get injured. So now, if I'm feeling like it's not happening, I'll tell Scott and we'll either lighten the intensity that day or even give it a miss. Looking back, although the time when I was struggling with glandular fever was really tough, it was undoubtedly a blessing in disguise. It forced me to really start listening to my body and, in doing this, I'm hoping to lengthen my career.

THE ROAD TO RIO

By taking time off and allowing my body to reboot, I came back fresh, strong and full of fight. In the build-up to Rio, I had loads of great routines and quality training in the bag and my confidence was really high. Going into the World Championships, I felt great and made British gymnastics history by becoming champion on the pommel and the first British male world champion. I still had to be aware of not pushing too hard, as at that time I was still doing all six pieces of kit, whereas now I just specialise on the pommel and floor. So I had to be really smart in my preparation and take days off when I needed them.

In the final build-up to Rio there was no avoiding ramping things up, though, and I did loads of what we call 'control competitions'. This basically involves simulating the demands of a major competition. It's really gruelling but is an essential part of preparation and I needed to know that I could cope with the schedule. During the Olympics, after the team final, I had two days before the all-round final. In the past I would have trained on those days but I felt absolutely shattered and said to Scott that I needed a day off. It was the first time I'd ever done this a day before a competition but my experience with glandular fever and the lessons I'd learned gave me the confidence to know that it was 100 per cent the right thing to do. It really paid off and I still have to pinch myself that I won those two gold medals and a bronze. I also believe that they had such a positive impact on the country, and there are plenty of great young gymnasts that I've met who were inspired by what I achieved and that makes me feel as proud as the medals do.

BACK TO NORMALITY (SORT OF)

Coming back to the UK was just surreal and I couldn't get over how fired up people were by the Olympics; the reception I got was just amazing. I took three months off from training, which was by far the longest amount of time I'd ever been away from the gym. I used the time to really appreciate what I'd achieved and to let it sink in. Scott and I had come up with a four-year plan to put me in a position to maybe win one gold medal, so to come home with two and a bronze took a bit of adjusting to. The time off also allowed me to go on holiday with Leah and to thank all the friends, family and sponsors who'd supported me.

Getting an MBE was a real surprise and going to Buckingham Palace to collect it was an amazing experience. I was really lucky that I received mine from the Queen herself, as she doesn't do it that often any more. She was either very well briefed or is a real gymnastics fan because she talked incredibly knowledgeably about the sport and how excited she was about how many people, especially children, had been inspired by our Olympic success. I must confess, I often forget I have the MBE but, when I think about it, having those three letters after my name is pretty cool and a huge honour.

I also squeezed in getting married. Leah and I met when I moved to South Essex when I was thirteen and we became an item when I was fourteen. She was a gymnast too and I think her having that understanding and first-hand experience of the sport really helps. She's been by my side for this whole mad journey and I know that without her there I would have really struggled, especially when things haven't gone quite to plan, which is an inevitability in sport. It makes us both laugh that it took ten years for us to get around to getting married but that's the reality of the constant cycle of training and competition; finding that window is really tough! Our wedding day was incredible. I thought I'd experienced some amazing highs at both London and Rio but, sitting on that top table with Leah looking so beautiful next to me and all of our friends and family there, it was a whole new level. If we could do it all again tomorrow, we definitely would!

BACK TO THE GYM

By the end of the three months I was itching to get back to the gym. Going into 2017, the plan was, despite being back in hard training, to take six months out from competition. The reasoning behind this was that Scott and I had set ourselves the massive target of not coming back to competition with any of the same routines that I'd performed in Rio. It was a really long time to not compete but it was necessary to allow me to make, practise and refine those upgrades. I wanted to have the hardest routine possible among my competitors so the result would simply be down to me executing it as cleanly as I could. Eventually, though, we had to unveil those routines and that was at the 2017 World Champs, where I'd be attempting to retain my title. I've never felt pressure like it, mostly from myself and because I was out of the routine of competition. There's also no doubt that with each year, and as routines get more challenging, competition gets harder on my body. However, this is balanced by experience, a more mature and efficient approach to training and the amazing people I have supporting me. It was a great feeling retaining that title and I felt a massive sense of relief. The signs were all good for 2018 and going into the lead-up to Tokyo, but I then suffered another dip.

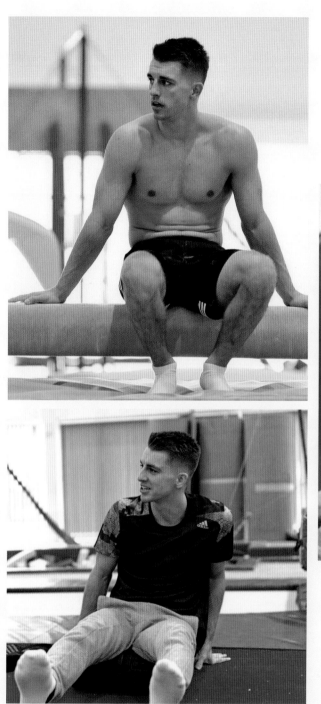

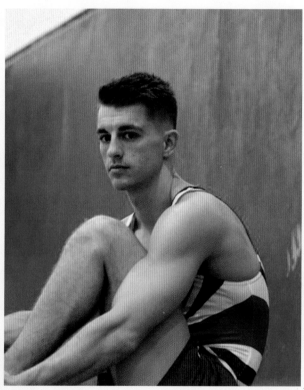

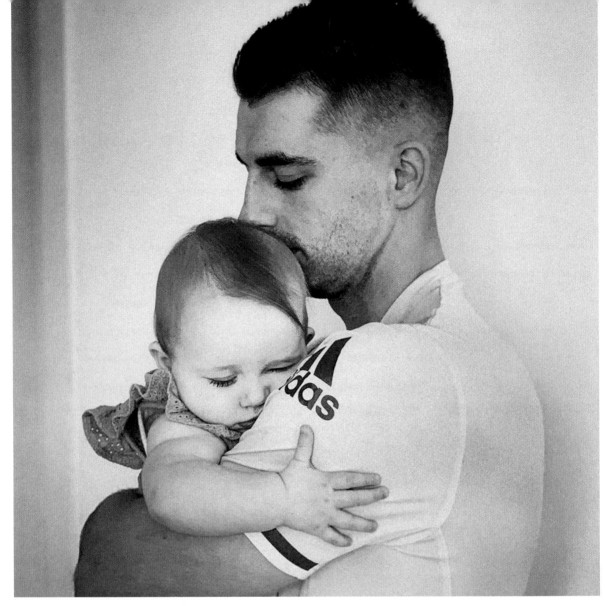

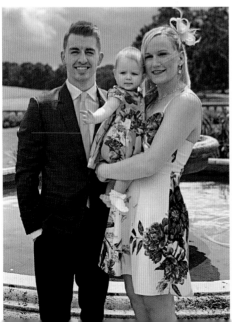

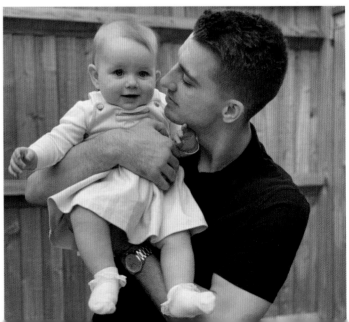

UNDER THE GLARE OF THE PUBLIC EYE

Looking back to the four years between London and Rio, the first two years were tough and I suffered a drop in my competition performances. The fact that a similar thing happened, although slightly delayed by my time off, after Rio shouldn't have been a surprise. Upgrading my routines was such a huge risk that mistakes were inevitable. A silver medal at the 2018 Europeans and the same at the Worlds shouldn't have felt like a disappointment – and if you'd offered me those results ten years ago I would have bitten your hand off – but, as an athlete, it did. I guess the big difference between post-London and post-Rio was that I was much more in the public eye. In the eyes of the media the Rio Golden Boy had failed, and those sorts of comments hurt. I'd try to explain it in interviews but going backwards short term to move forwards in the long term can be quite a hard concept to get across.

It actually spurred me on, especially when people started suggesting the possibility of retirement. There were a lot of people who said that, in my place, they would have gone out on a high after Rio but I felt, and still feel, that I've got loads more to get out of gymnastics and a lot more to give. There's no way I'm ready to stop and I feel like I'm improving each year. More than anything else, I still love what I'm doing and feel excited every day I go to the gym. I know that I can still deliver the results and give more back to the sport that has been so good to me. By training smart and staying fit and injury free, I'd like to do two more Olympics.

BACK TO MY BEST AND A NEW ADDITION

Coming into 2019, I felt like I had to back up what I'd been saying the previous year and deliver on the plan. I also felt like I had to put in a big performance at the Europeans. When I won the title comfortably it was a massive relief. I'm aware it sounds as though this is the case with every title, and it's true to an extent, but winning is usually combined with equal joy and disbelief. But this title was empowerment for me, as it put that year of publicly perceived failure and disappointment behind me.

What was pure, undiluted joy, though, was the birth of my daughter, Willow. I know it sounds like a horrendous cliché, but when I first held Willow it was the proudest moment of my life, along with my wedding day. Forget winning Olympic and world titles! Parenthood has been pretty mad and full-on. Leah and I are both fairly young and it still feels surreal to think that we're parents. Every small milestone in Willow's development – her rolling over, smiling or laughing – seems like the biggest thing in the world to us. It's given us both perspective about what's really important and that has actually had a hugely beneficial effect on my gymnastics. It has sort of taken the pressure off and I know, even if a session at the gym doesn't quite go according to plan, Leah and Willow are at home to make it all better. Less pressure means I'm more relaxed and I'm performing better, so it's win-win! I was a bit concerned before Willow was born about my sleep: I've always been used to getting 10–11 hours each night because that amount of good-quality sleep is crucial to my recovery from workouts. Fortunately, though, she seems to have inherited my love of sleep and, touch wood, she's super easy-going. As I'm writing this, she's eight months old and the time is just flying by. I had three competitions and a major event within her first month but she's been here, there and everywhere with us and taken it all in her stride.

I'm so excited about showing her the world and what I do, and I really want her to see and remember me competing live and not just on YouTube. I was so proud to regain the world title on the pommel at the 2019 World Championships in October and bring my medal back home to show Willow and Leah. The prospect of having Willow in the crowd at Tokyo 2020 is an amazing thought and a real added incentive to be at those Games.

WRITING A BOOK

For a while now I've wanted to pass on some of the knowledge about health and fitness that I've acquired throughout my career so far, making it relevant for the general population. I find it staggering and really scary that so many people get out of breath climbing the stairs, or can't jump up on a bench in the park or play a game of football with their kids. People just aren't making the most of the incredible potential of their bodies and, although I'm not for one moment suggesting that everyone can or should be an Olympic gymnast, I really believe that anyone can benefit from gymnastic-style training. It provides such a brilliant foundation in terms of mobility, body control and strength and, as it's largely based around bodyweight exercises, it can be done practically anywhere.

WORKOUTS

I was lucky enough to test the water with some of my ideas and routines with a DFS campaign supporting the British Heart Foundation. They went down really well, and I got some great feedback that spurred me on with my idea for a book. Having had my own experience of illness through overtraining, I want to encourage sustainable lifestyle changes through manageable and progressive workouts, rather than through an exercise binge that promises results within an unrealistic timescale. This isn't a 'get fit quick' book. However, my 15–30 minute workouts are easy to integrate into your life, require no expensive kit or gym membership and will address all aspects of your fitness using exercises that I've been doing myself from the age of seven – and still do now.

RECIPES

Similarly, when it comes to nutrition, I have steered clear of faddy diets and complicated recipes. I really don't like the word 'diet' as it implies a short-term fix rather than a permanent change. Small and sustainable changes towards healthier eating will always trump short-term and overly drastic dietary interventions. Healthy eating doesn't have to be boring and you don't have to feel as though you're missing out on treats. Many of my recipes are healthy twists on junk-food favourites and are all super easy to cook.

By combining my no-frills and fad-free approach to nutrition with my fun and effective workouts, you'll unlock your body's true potential – and maybe even discover your inner gymnast.

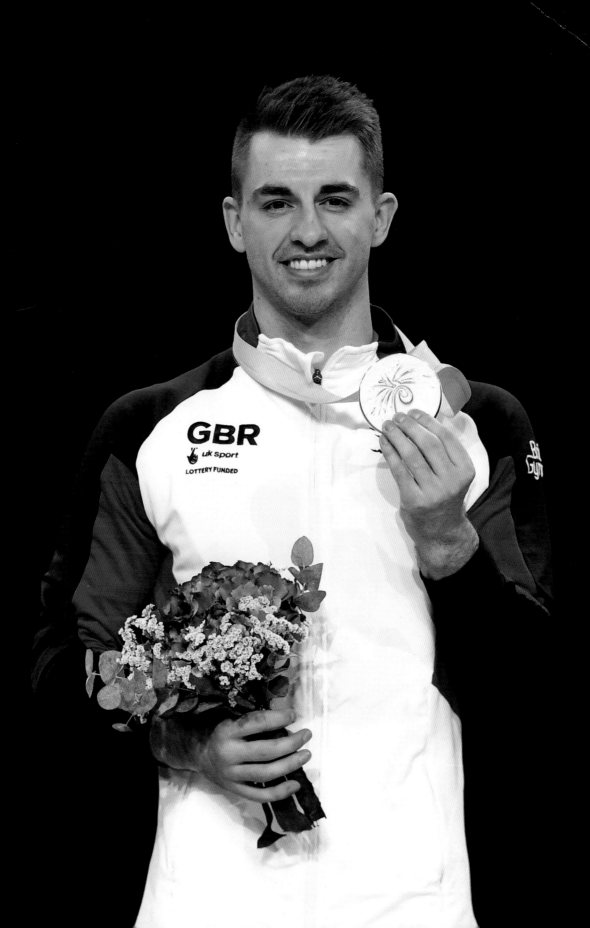

GIVING GYMNASTICS A GO

The workouts in this book are 100 per cent based on the exercises I've been doing from the age of seven and they are still a part of my workout routines. They have given me the conditioning foundations that have allowed me to develop and perfect the advanced skills and routines I now perform. I still do them because they keep my joints strong and mobile, protecting me against injury, especially as I get older.

If you're already involved in gymnastics, you'll soon realise how beneficial my workouts are for your performance. However, I'm also hoping that, along with noticing the benefits to your overall health and appearance, some of you might be inspired to give gymnastics a go. It doesn't matter what age you are, anyone can try it. Leah and I are very proud to have created Max Whitlock Gymnastics classes to provide more opportunities for young people to enjoy, in my view, the best sport in the world. Many clubs offer classes for all age groups and abilities. Get in touch with a club in your area for more information.

Many people are put off by gymnastics because they see what top-level gymnasts do and are scared or intimidated. The key thing to know is you'll learn gymnastic skills in an incredibly safe environment with soft crash mats, foam pits and, most importantly, great coaches. No one goes straight into attempting a somersault. There are probably ten stages and progressions to work through before you're ready for one.

There's a great social side to gymnastics, too. At my training sessions, I obviously train hard but I always have a laugh with the group of guys I train with. We'll joke, kick a football about and encourage each other. It makes the hard work seem easier and is definitely one of the main reasons why I love my sport.

I genuinely believe that gymnastics gives kids a brilliant foundation, whether they carry it on as they get older or gravitate towards other sports. It develops all-round strength, mobility and body awareness. The latter is especially useful in all sports because it teaches you how to fall and land safely. Willow is already in a baby gymnastics class so that she can start to develop these foundations but I'm keen for her to be involved in as many sports as possible.

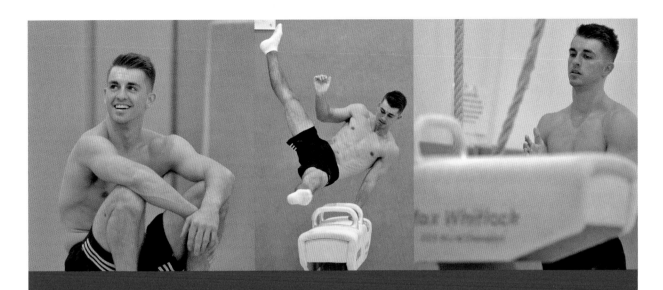

'IT DOESN'T MATTER WHAT AGE YOU ARE, ANYONE CAN TRY IT.'

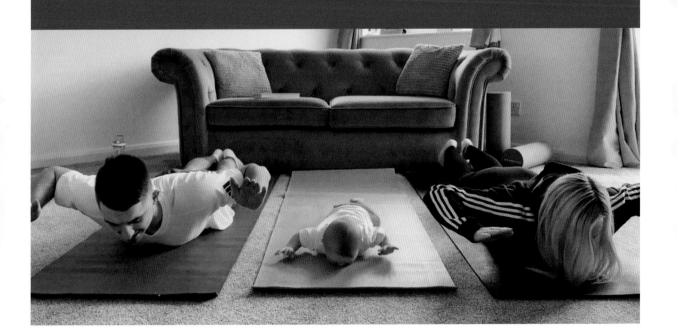

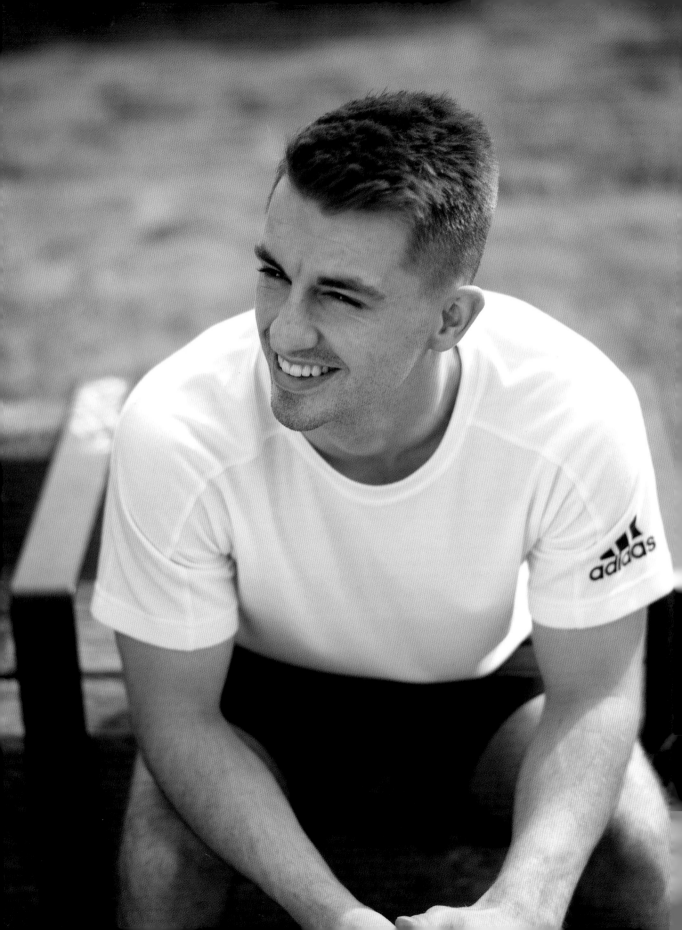

GENERAL WORKOUT GUIDELINES
FOR SOFA, CUSHION CRUSHER
AND TOTAL BODY WORKOUTS

WHERE DO I START?

Even if you're already a regular exerciser, I would strongly suggest starting with the Level 1 Sofa and Cushion Crusher workouts (pages 45 and 65) as, unless you come from a gymnastic background, you'll likely find the movements challenging, especially maintaining them for 30 seconds. They also build the foundations of strength and mobility for the more demanding routines that follow.

For your first go, aim for two cycles through but, if that feels too easy, crack on for a third or maybe even a fourth.

HOW OFTEN SHOULD I WORK OUT?

You should aim to do these workouts at least three times per week but no more than every other day. You can stick to one workout or mix and match them. On 'off-days' there is no reason why you can't do my Stretching/Recovery Routine (page 144) or another complementary form of exercise. This could be something cardiovascular, such as running, cycling or swimming.

HOW DO I PROGRESS?

As the workouts use time rather than repetitions, they're effectively self-progressing. Each time you do an exercise, you're looking to do as many quality reps as you can within the 30 seconds, rather than a set number. Once you feel you're working strongly for all of the 30-second exercise blocks for 2 cycles through a Level 1 Sofa or

Cushion Crusher workout, add another cycle and keep building in this way to 3 or 4 cycles.

Then you can move on to Level 2 Sofa or Cushion Crusher workouts (pages 50 and 71), going back down to 2 cycles initially and then building up again to 3 or 4 before moving on to Level 3.

You shouldn't try to rush through the levels. It's far better to spend a few sessions consolidating a lower level routine rather than poorly executing one that's currently a bit too much for you.

Once you're maxing out with the Level 3 Sofa or Cushion Crusher Workouts (pages 56 and 77) and are finding 3–4 cycles and 30-second exercise blocks relatively easy, you'll have achieved a very high level of overall fitness; I still find these workouts tough! You can then move on to the challenges of the Total Body Workouts (page 86) and work through the 3 levels in the same way.

The progression from the Total Body Workouts is to my Home Bar Workouts (page 106), Rings Workouts (page 118) and finally, the ultimate challenge, my Perfect 10 Pro Park Workouts (page 126). The structure of these workouts is different to the previous ones so make sure you thoroughly read their specific instructions. **Don't rush to attempt these workouts.** It's only with the excellent foundations of fitness that consistent completion of the previous workouts will give you, that you'll get the most from these more advanced workouts and be able to complete them safely and effectively.

EXAMPLE TRAINING WEEKS

Here are some examples of how you could construct your training week based on the guidelines described above. As you can see there's plenty of scope for flexibility and moving things about to fit in with your life. Don't try to pack in too much, as more isn't always more, consistency is key and recovery allows your body to adapt and become stronger.

BEGINNER TRAINING WEEK

MONDAY	TUESDAY	WEDNESDAY	THURSDAY	FRIDAY	SATURDAY	SUNDAY
Sofa Workout Level 1 (See page 45)	Rest	Cushion Crusher Level 1 (See page 65)	Rest	Sofa Workout Level 1 (See page 45)	Swimming	Stretching/ Recovery Routine (See page 144)

INTERMEDIATE TRAINING WEEK

MONDAY	TUESDAY	WEDNESDAY	THURSDAY	FRIDAY	SATURDAY	SUNDAY
Sofa Workout Level 3 (See page 56)	Stretching/ Recovery Routine (See page 144)	Cushion Crusher Level 3 (See page 77)	Rest	Total Body Workout Level 1 (See page 87)	Running	Stretching/ Recovery Routine (See page 144)

ADVANCED TRAINING WEEK

MONDAY	TUESDAY	WEDNESDAY	THURSDAY	FRIDAY	SATURDAY	SUNDAY
Total Body Workout Level 3 (See page 98)	Stretching/ Recovery Routine (See page 144)	Cushion Crusher Level 3 (See page 77)	Stretching/ Recovery Routine (See page 144)	Rings Workout Level 1 (See page 119)	Stretching/ Recovery Routine (See page 144)	Rest

WARMING UP AND COOLING DOWN

Before a workout, always spend 5–10 minutes following my 5-minute Pre-workout Warm-up Routine. You should feel warm, maybe sweating slightly, and be ready to go.

Don't forget to cool down. If you're short of time, follow my 5-minute Post-workout Stretch Routine or, for a deeper stretch, work through my Stretching/Recovery Routine. You can also do my Foam Roller Routine post workout.

STRUCTURE

The Sofa, Cushion Crusher and Total Body Workouts all use the same simple-to-follow structure:

Each cycle will take approximately 4 minutes. Therefore, the total time for a workout, including warm-up and cool-down, will be approximately 20–30 minutes.

There are typically 6 exercises per cycle: 2 lower body, 2 mid-section/core and 2 upper body.

You work for 30 seconds per exercise; use a countdown timer on your phone. You're looking to do as many reps as possible in that time but without rushing the movement and without sacrificing good form. You'll find, with some of the exercises, that working slower with more control is actually more intense. Some of the exercises are static holds and, in those cases, you're looking to maintain strong form for the entire 30 seconds.

Take a short 10-second breather between exercises.

Take a longer 1-minute rest between cycles.

You should aim to complete a minimum of 2 cycles per workout but you can do 3 cycles or more depending on your fitness level and available time.

TECHNIQUE TIPS

Take a moment before doing a workout for the first time to make sure you're familiar and comfortable with the exercises; you'll get a far better quality workout if you do this.

Don't forget to breathe! For dynamic movements, such as squats, breathe out on the effort/lift and in on the lower/relax. For static holds, such as planks and bridges, try to breathe in a relaxed and controlled manner.

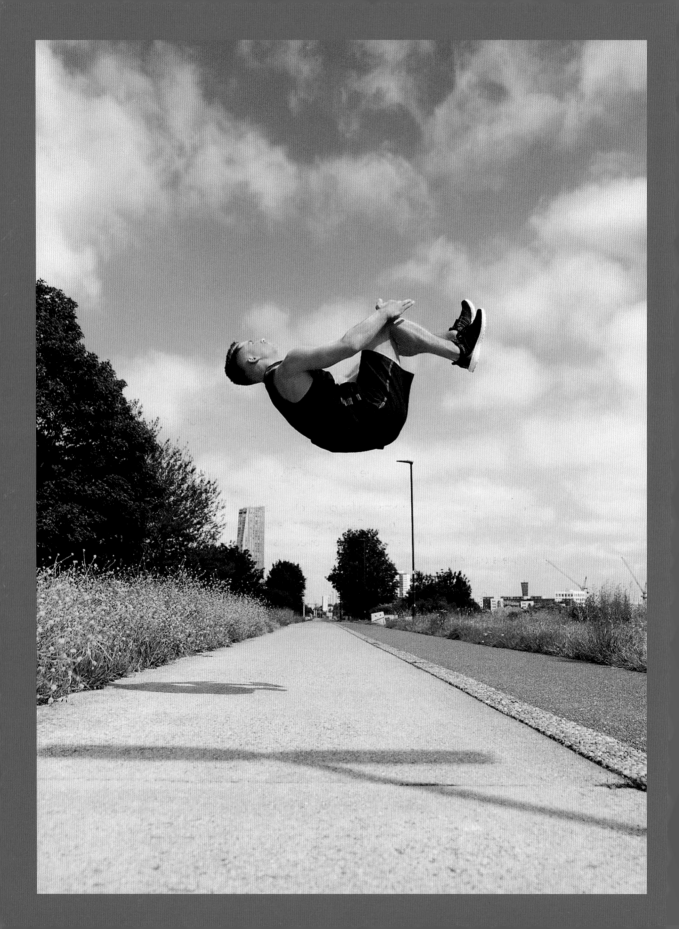

MAX'S LIFE:
MY TRAINING

At this current stage in my career, if I'm not in the run-up to a competition, my training is about consistency, keeping my fitness at a good level and my skills ticking over. My actual hours in the gym remain pretty constant at 20–25 hours per week. In the lead-up to a competition, though, I'll have a 2–3 month build where the intensity of what I'm doing will increase within those hours. It's all about developing the fitness to allow me to get through an entire routine.

On weekdays I'll typically train between 1100-1500. Mondays, Wednesdays and Fridays are my slightly easier days. Tuesdays and Thursdays are my harder 'routine days' where we'll be practising for competitions and loading the workout up in terms of volume and intensity. Saturdays are a competition run-through, where I'll try to simulate the demands of an event as closely as possible, and Sundays are a day off.

Every day in the gym is fairly similar and, although this might appear to be monotonous, it's all about routine and, the more of a routine I can get into, the better. At the end of the day, when I go into competitions, I'm performing routines so, if everything both inside and outside the gym are routines, that works best for me.

If you're going to take one thing from my training and apply it to your own, it will be establishing and setting in stone your own routine. You've got to prioritise your training, ink it into your diary and make it something that can't be bumped. The joy of my workouts in this book is that they're incredibly time-efficient but you still need to commit to that time and not have it just floating as a maybe. You'll soon find, if you commit to that 20–30 minutes regularly, it'll become your routine, a habit and second nature.

5-MINUTE PRE-WORKOUT WARM-UP ROUTINE

This 5-minute warm-up is the minimum I'd recommend doing before starting a workout. If you feel you want to do longer, you can work through it multiple times, extend the Heart Rate Raiser at the start or even do some more extensive cardiovascular training, such as cycling, running or rowing, beforehand. The key is that you should feel warm, mobilised and ready to go.

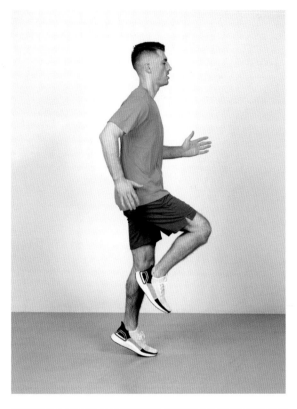

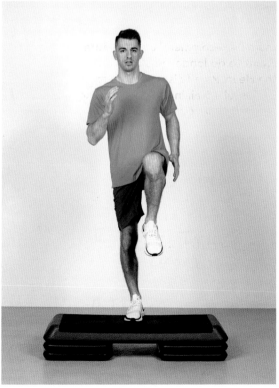

1. HEART RATE RAISER (3 MINUTES)

To progressively elevate your heart rate and to raise your body temperature.

March or jog on the spot. Use a bottom stair or bench for some step-ups, try skipping or mix things up.

Start at an easy intensity and try to build it progressively over the 3 minutes.

By the end of the 3 minutes you should be breathing quite hard, feeling warmer and maybe starting to sweat a bit.

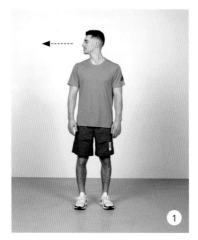

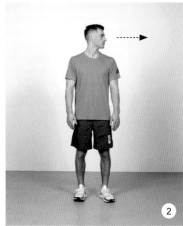

2. NECK ROLLS
(30 SECONDS)

Starting to warm up your head and neck.

Begin by looking from side to side. Progress to chin to chest and then looking up at the ceiling.

As your neck loosens, move on to full circles, working in both directions.

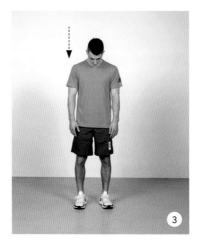

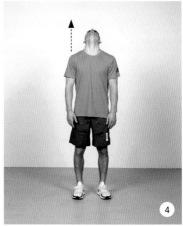

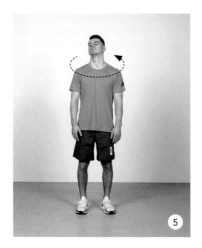

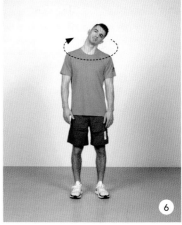

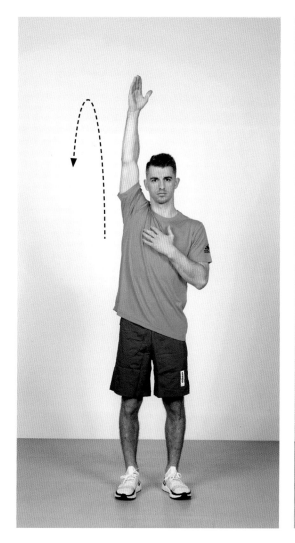
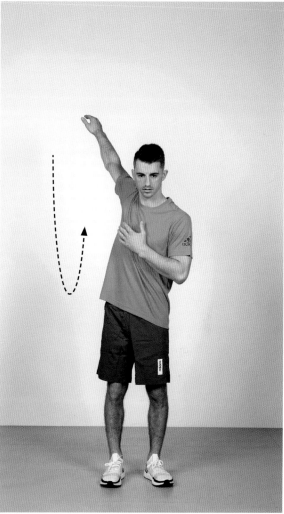

3. SINGLE ARM SWINGS (15 SECONDS EACH ARM)

Moving on to your arms, shoulders and chest.

Swing one arm in wide smooth circles, trying to brush your ear with your shoulder.

Start in whichever direction, forwards or backwards, feels most natural to you but switch once things start to loosen up.

Change arms and repeat.

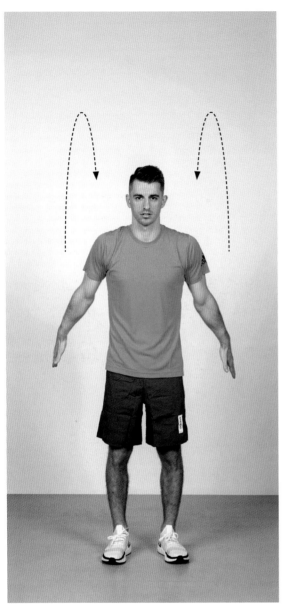
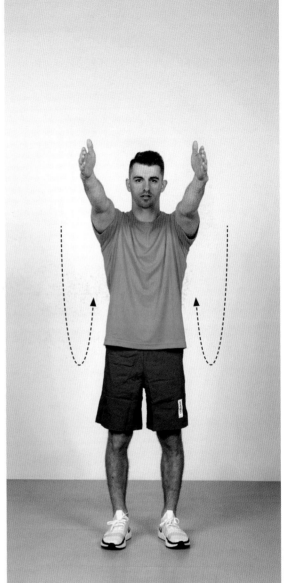

4. DOUBLE ARM SWINGS (30 SECONDS)

Progressing from the Single Arm Swings.

Again, start in whichever direction feels easier and then switch halfway through the time.

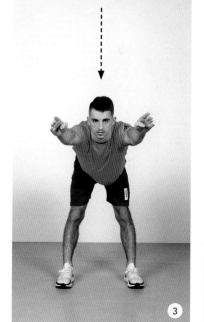

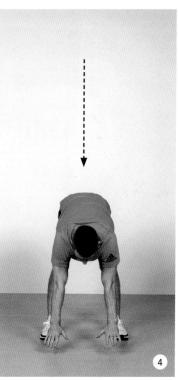

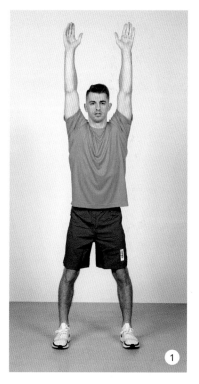

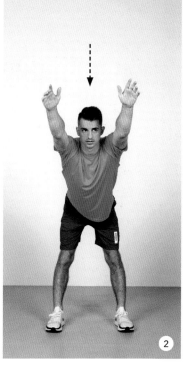

5. REACH UP AND DROP DOWN (30 SECONDS)

A great mobilisation movement for the whole body.

Reach up to the ceiling, trying to stretch out your entire body and make yourself as tall as possible.

Pause briefly.

Fold at the waist and, trying to maintain a neutral spine and straight but not locked legs, reach down towards the floor.

Pause briefly, feeling a stretch develop in your hamstrings and lower back. See if you can go a little lower but avoid bouncing.

Come back up. Keep repeating the movement, trying to get a bit higher and a bit lower each time. In 30 seconds, you should get through 3–5 cycles.

6. BOUNCING ON THE SPOT (30 SECONDS)

Getting your heart rate up again and a chance to shake everything out.

With soft knees and staying up on the balls of your feet, bounce on the spot.

Try to minimise your contact time with the floor, imagine you're on a hot tin roof!

Shake your arms out as you bounce.

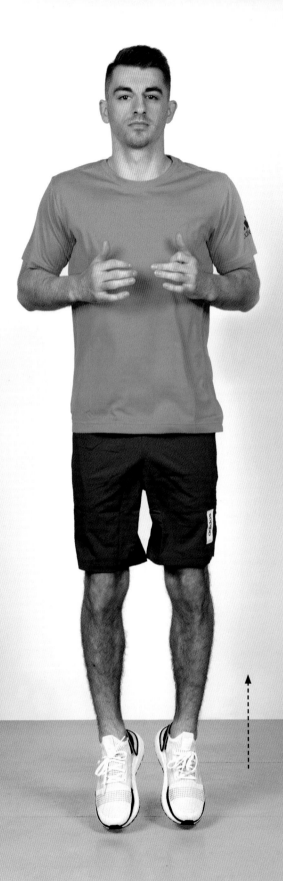

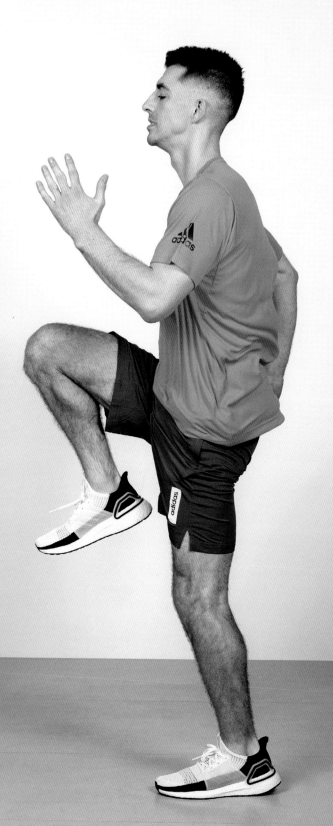

7. SPRINTING ON THE SPOT (30 SECONDS)

Taking your heart rate even higher and a final blast before hitting the workout.

Sprint on the spot, aiming to bring your knees up to waist height.

Pump your arms.

Get up on your toes and think fast feet.

5-MINUTE POST-WORKOUT STRETCH ROUTINE

HOLD EACH STRETCH FOR AROUND 30 SECONDS
TAKE YOUR TIME WITHIN EACH STRETCH

Like with warming up, 5 minutes is the minimum I'd recommend for stretching after your workout but, if you can, dedicating a bit more time will be beneficial. You can either repeat the routine or hold each position for longer. Or, for a really deep stretch, do my full Stretching/Recovery Routine (page 144). Try to relax, breathe deeply, allow the stretch to develop and deepen but don't bounce. You could even finish the routine by simply lying down, focusing on your breath and maybe trying some meditation.

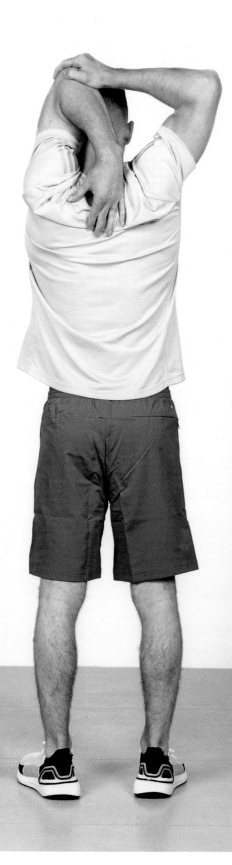

1. ARM OVER HEAD

Stretching out the backs of your arms (triceps), which will have worked hard during any pushing or pressing movements.

Standing, kneeling or sitting, extend one arm above your head and then bend it and reach down to between your shoulder blades.

Hold the elbow of that arm with your other hand and gently pull inwards and push downwards to intensify the stretch.

Repeat with the other arm.

2. CHEST STRETCH

Focusing on your chest (pecs), and front of your shoulders.

Lie on your stomach on the floor with one arm bent at 90 degrees.

With the other hand, push away from the floor.

You should feel a stretch across your chest and shoulder of your extended arm.

Repeat on the other side.

3. SEAL STRETCH

Brilliant for your lower back but will also help your abdominal muscles (abs) recover from sit-up-type movements and stretch your hips and thighs.

Lie face down as if you're going to perform a press-up.

Straighten your arms to raise your chest but don't allow your groin and legs to come off the ground.

Actively push your groin and legs down as your upper body comes up to create an arch in your lower back.

If this feels too intense, just come up onto your elbows.

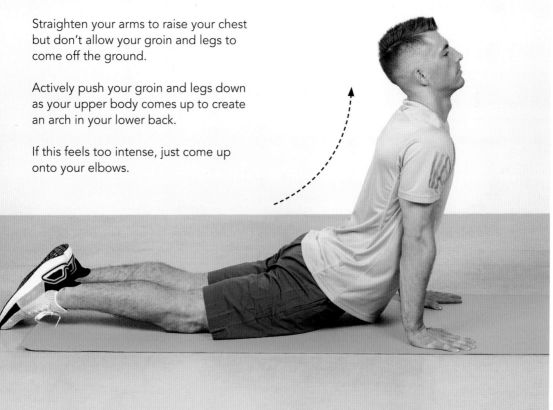

4. KNEELING LUNGE

A deep stretch for the front of your thighs (quads) and hip flexors.

From a kneeling position, bring one leg forwards so that you're in a kneeling lunge. You may find it more comfortable if your other knee is on a cushion.

Make sure the knee of your front leg is directly over the ankle and that your upper body is tall with your centre of gravity over your kneeling knee.

Contract your trunk muscles and squeeze your backside (glutes) to create a stretch in the hip and thigh of your kneeling leg.

Allow the stretch to develop and intensify by sliding your front foot further forwards.

Repeat with the other leg.

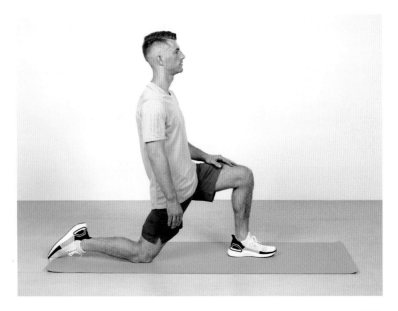

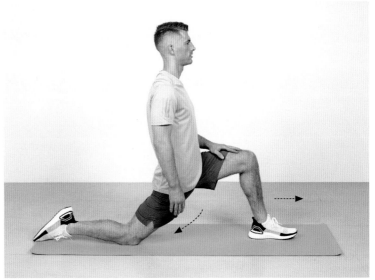

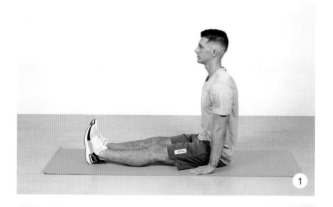

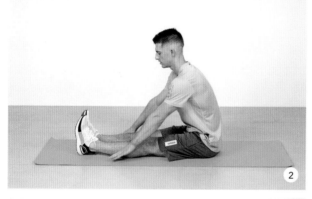

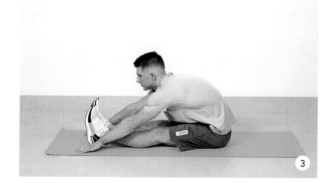

5. SIT AND REACH

Increasing flexibility in the backs of your legs (hamstrings) and lower back.

Sit on the floor with straight legs.

Keeping your head and chest up and avoiding rounding your back, lean forwards from your waist, creeping your hands down your shins towards your feet.

When you feel a stretch in your hamstrings, pause, allow it to ease and then creep forwards a bit more.

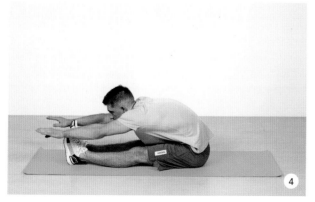

WHY DO I NEED TO WARM-UP AND COOL-DOWN?

WARM-UP

Warming up is essential to prepare your body and mind to perform at their very best. Whether in day-to-day training or competing in an Olympic final, I won't just go straight into a demanding routine. I'll go through a thorough warm-up that prepares me both physically and mentally for the exertions to come.

A warm-up results in a number of physiological responses that are essential for optimal performance. A good analogy is it being a good idea to allow your car engine to warm up on a cold day. Fuel and oil become more viscous and flow better. Moving parts glide past each other more smoothly and the whole engine performs far more efficiently than if you'd just pressed the accelerator to the floor immediately.

Your heart rate should be increased progressively, enabling more oxygen to be transported through your blood to, and used within, the working muscles. With increased body temperature, the range of motion around your joints will also improve and you will get close to your optimal efficiency very quickly. These responses mean that you'll be able to perform the workout better, get more from the exercises and reduce the risk of injury.

Having a structured warm-up routine that you're familiar with will also help to get you in the right mindset for a workout. The routine will quickly become second nature and you'll find that doing it will act as an 'on' switch for you.

COOL-DOWN

A cool-down effectively reverses the process and helps return your body and mind to their pre-exercise state. It will aid recovery and the fitness gains you'll get from the workout. It should be viewed as the first step to preparing your body for your next training session, the day ahead or just relaxing. A cool-down also allows you to mentally wind down after a hard workout and gives you time to reflect on your performance.

A cool-down will help remove metabolic waste products from your muscles that build up during training. If you don't cool down, these metabolites will 'sit' there and potentially inhibit recovery. A cool-down will also minimise the likelihood of you feeling dizzy, nauseous or fainting post exercise. It will also allow your blood to redistribute around the body.

The stretching and flexibility work you'll do in the cool-down address a heightened sensitivity in your muscles to ranges of movement beyond those which you experience during your regular life. This heightened sensitivity, if left unaddressed, can easily lead to imbalances, poor muscle function and potentially pain or injury. Also, as many of the movements in the workouts focus on flexibility and mobility, if you can improve your range of motion, you'll get more out of them.

SOFA WORKOUTS

4 MINUTES PER CYCLE
2–4 CYCLES
30 SECONDS EACH EXERCISE
10 SECONDS REST BETWEEN EXERCISES
1 MINUTE REST BETWEEN CYCLES

The great thing about these Sofa Workouts is that you can do them anywhere. At home, in a hotel room, in the park or even in the gym. As long as you have a sofa, bed or bench you'll be able to get an effective workout.

They're incredibly time-efficient and, even with a warm-up, cool-down and 3 cycles through the routine, you'll be done in under 25 minutes. Remember, you're doing each exercise for 30 seconds and trying to do as many quality reps as possible. Work as fast as you can but don't sacrifice form or technique.

SOFA WORKOUT – LEVEL 1

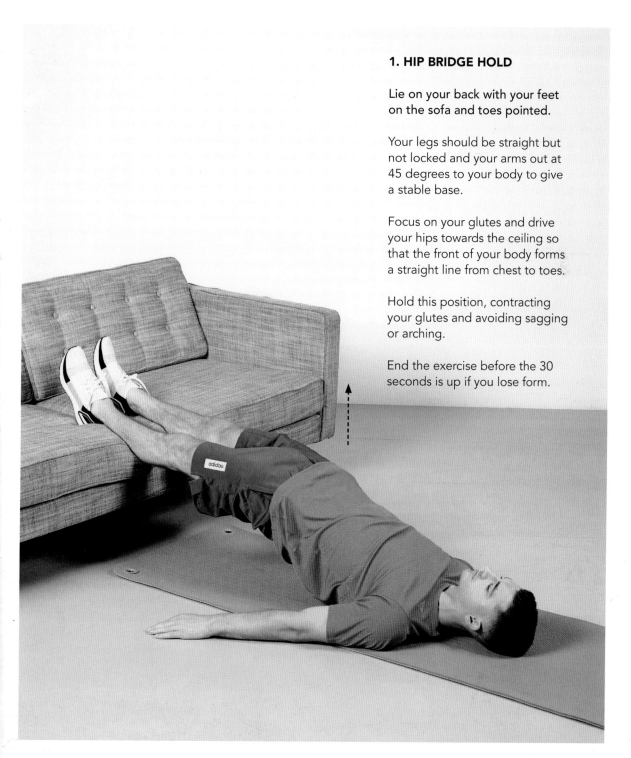

1. HIP BRIDGE HOLD

Lie on your back with your feet on the sofa and toes pointed.

Your legs should be straight but not locked and your arms out at 45 degrees to your body to give a stable base.

Focus on your glutes and drive your hips towards the ceiling so that the front of your body forms a straight line from chest to toes.

Hold this position, contracting your glutes and avoiding sagging or arching.

End the exercise before the 30 seconds is up if you lose form.

2. LAZY SQUATS

Don't be fooled by the 'lazy', as these work the whole of the lower body and will get your heart and lungs working too.

Sit on the sofa with your feet and knees approximately hip width apart. Your heels should be close to, or touching, the sofa and your toes pointing slightly outwards.

With your arms out in front of you and keeping your head up, stand up.

With control, sit back down and repeat.

Avoid allowing your knees to collapse in towards each other as you stand.

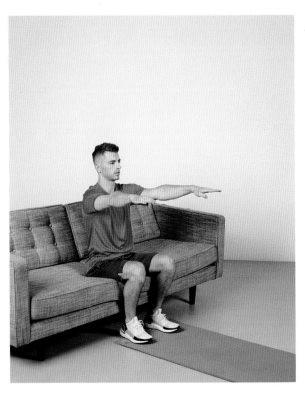

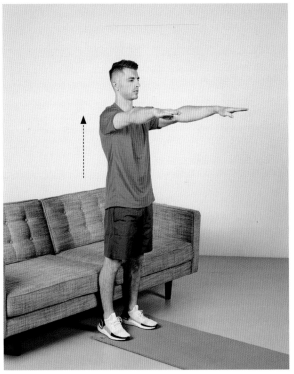

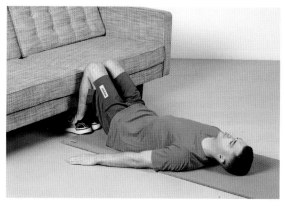

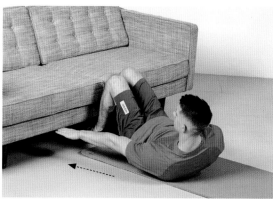

3. SOFA SIDE TOUCHES

This movement targets your abs, especially the obliques; there's also a mobility component.

Lie on your back with your knees bent, toes tucked under the sofa and arms out to the side.

Contract your abdominals to bring your torso slightly off the floor. Try to push your lower back into the floor as you do this.

Holding this position, work from side to side (imagine a penguin walking!), aiming to touch the sofa on each side. If you can't quite reach, don't worry, just go as far as you can while maintaining form.

4. PLANK ON ELBOWS

Planks are one of the most functional and effective core-strengthening exercises you can do and the strength you'll develop by doing them will lay the foundations for more advanced movements.

Adopt a position with your elbows on the sofa, approximately shoulder width apart and hands interlaced in front of you. Your feet are on the floor and you're up on your toes.

Keep the body straight (you're a 'plank') and brace through your core by consciously tensing your abs.

Hold the position, avoiding arching or sagging.

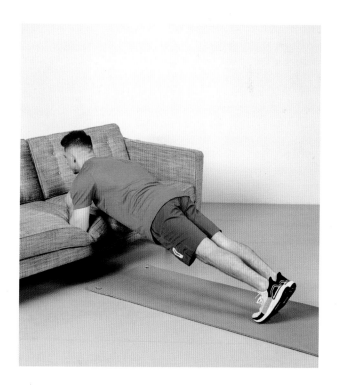

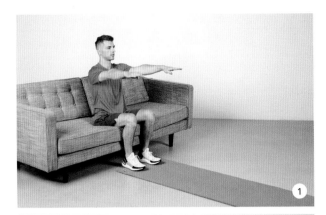

5. SITTING TO CATERPILLAR WALK TO FRONT SUPPORT

A total body strength and mobility exercise.

Sit on the sofa with your feet and knees approximately hip width apart. Your heels should be close to, or touching, the sofa, your toes pointing slightly outwards and arms out in front of you.

Rocking forwards, drop your chest towards your knees and come off the sofa, reaching your hands down onto the floor.

Walk forwards with your hands until you're fully extended in a press-up position; no arching or sagging.

Walk back with your hands, return to the seated start position and repeat.

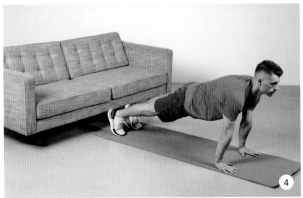

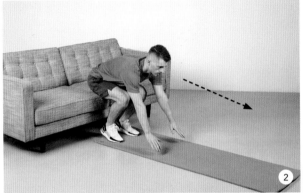

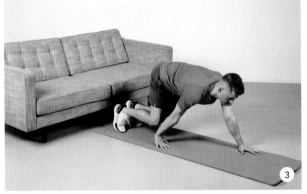

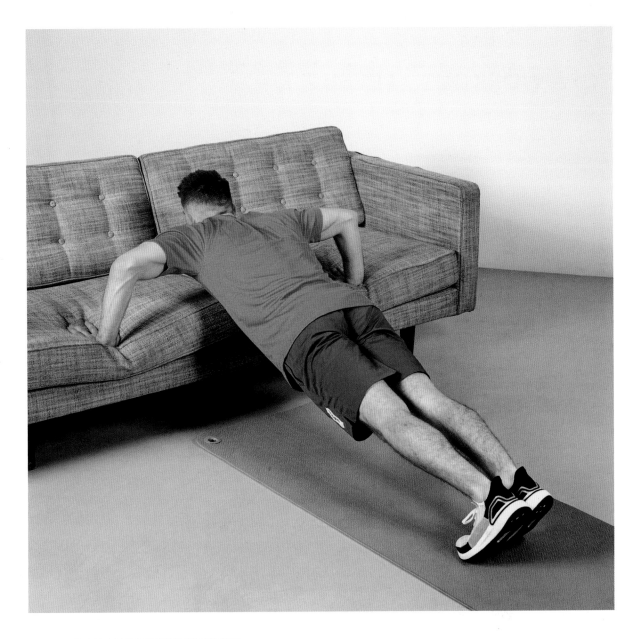

6. WIDE ARM PRESS-UP HOLD

As well as developing trunk strength, this exercise will also open up your chest, which is important if you spend a lot of time working at a desk.

With your hands on the sofa wider than shoulder width apart, lower your chest towards the sofa to a depth where your upper arms are parallel to the sofa; you should feel a stretch/tension across your chest.

Hold the position avoiding any arching or sagging of your body.

SOFA WORKOUT – LEVEL 2

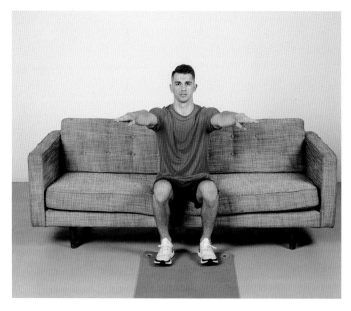

1. SOFA SQUAT JUMPS

A progression from the Lazy Squats (page 46) that'll develop explosive lower body strength and power, and challenge your cardiovascular system.

Start in the same squat position as the Lazy Squats.

Explode upwards, looking to jump as high as you can.

Land with soft knees, sink back down to touch the sofa with your backside but don't actually fully sit, and then jump again.

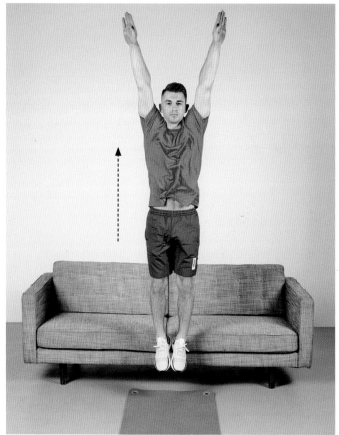

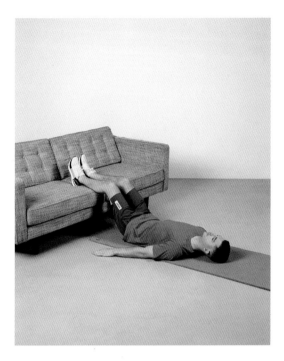

2. HIP BRIDGE BICYCLES

A more challenging variation of the Hip Bridge Hold (page 45) that brings in movement and single-legged bracing.

Get into a Hip Bridge Hold and, once stable, begin cycling your legs by bringing your knees alternately towards your chest.

Keep your hips up and try to avoid rocking them from side to side as you cycle.

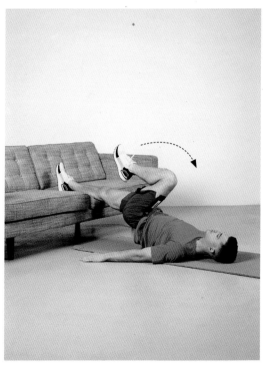

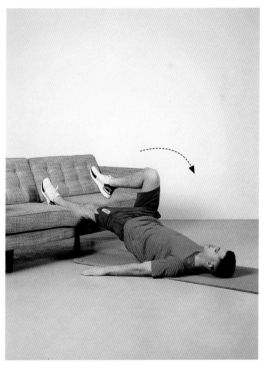

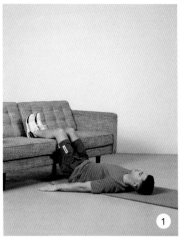
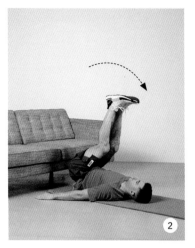
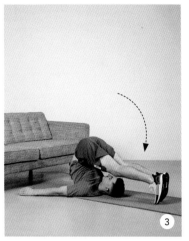

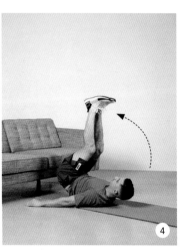
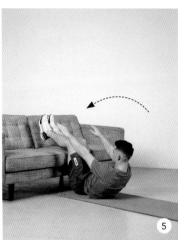
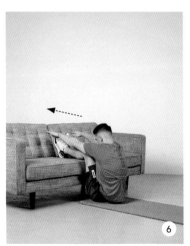

3. SIT-UP ROLL BACKS

Taking traditional sit-ups to a new level with added strength and mobility benefits.

Lie on the floor with your legs bent at 90 degrees and elevated on the sofa. Your backside should be close to, or touching, the sofa and your arms at 45 degrees to your body.

Swing your legs off the sofa and over your head, straightening them and lifting your backside off the floor.

Aim to touch the floor with your toes behind your head.

Roll back to the start position and, as your legs come back to the sofa, sit up and bring your knees to your chest and reach beyond your toes.

Lower back down to the floor and keep repeating the movement in a fluid but controlled manner.

4. TUCK DISH ON EDGE OF SOFA

A real test of abdominal strength and balance.

Sit on the edge of the sofa and, holding your arms out to aid balance and tensing your stomach muscles, lift your legs up and lean back.

You'll find a balance 'sweet-spot' where your abs are working really hard. Hold it there.

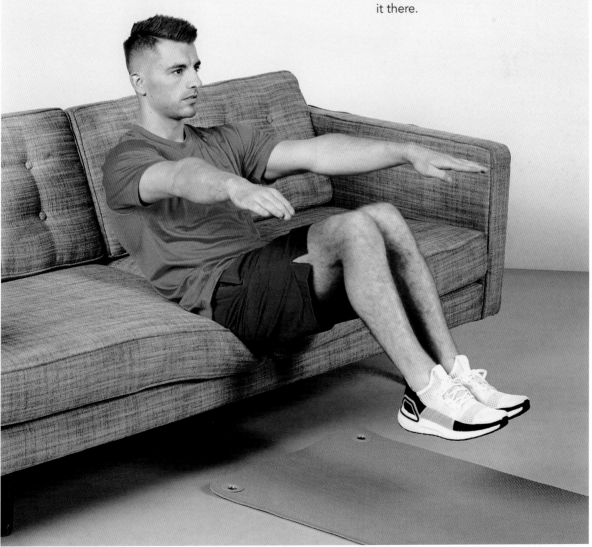

5. FRONT SUPPORT TO PIKE HANDSTAND

The pike movement is a gymnastic staple; you'll really feel it challenging your hamstring flexibility.

Start in a press-up hold position with your feet elevated on the sofa.

Pushing back through your hands, drive your backside up towards the ceiling.

Return to start position and repeat.

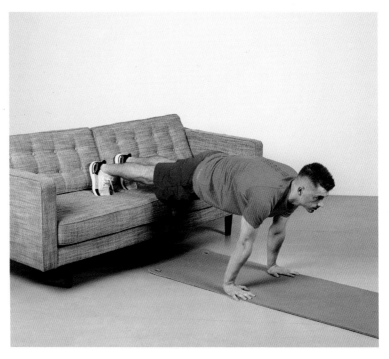

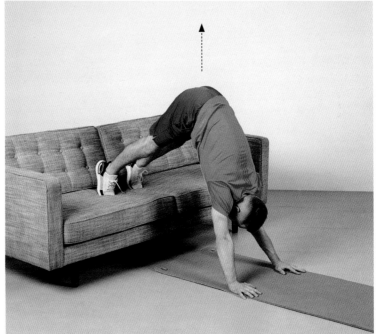

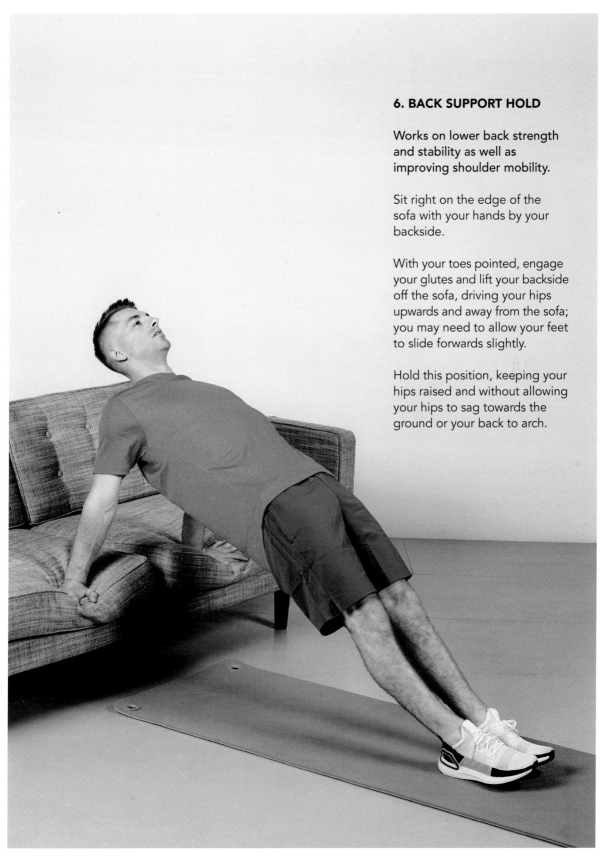

6. BACK SUPPORT HOLD

Works on lower back strength and stability as well as improving shoulder mobility.

Sit right on the edge of the sofa with your hands by your backside.

With your toes pointed, engage your glutes and lift your backside off the sofa, driving your hips upwards and away from the sofa; you may need to allow your feet to slide forwards slightly.

Hold this position, keeping your hips raised and without allowing your hips to sag towards the ground or your back to arch.

SOFA WORKOUT – LEVEL 3

1. SINGLE-LEGGED SOFA SQUATS

An extremely challenging squat variation that, along with being excellent for lower body strengthening, is also great for balance.

Set up as for a Lazy Squat (page 46) but stand using one leg, extending the other leg out in front of you.

Come right up onto your toes to really challenge your balance, then sit back down with control.

Change legs and repeat.

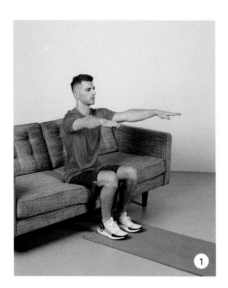

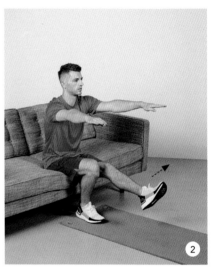

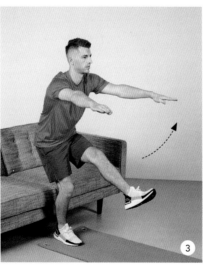

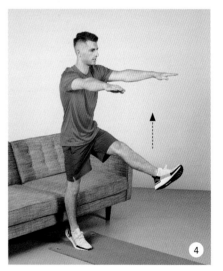

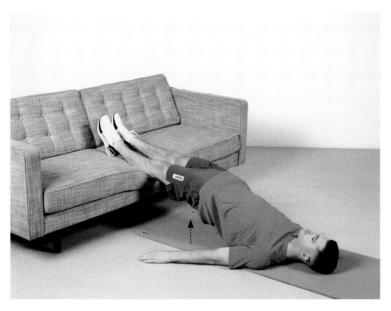

2. HIP BRIDGE SINGLE LEG LIFTS

Another Hip Bridge progression, bringing in straight-leg lifts which demand good hamstring flexibility.

From a Hip Bridge Hold position (page 45), keeping both legs straight, raise one, aiming for a 90-degree angle to the other leg.

Lower the leg with control and lightly touch the sofa with your calf.

Perform three reps with one leg, change to the other, perform another three reps and keep alternating in this way.

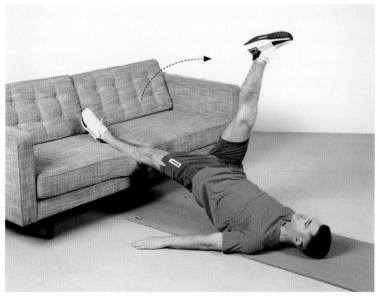

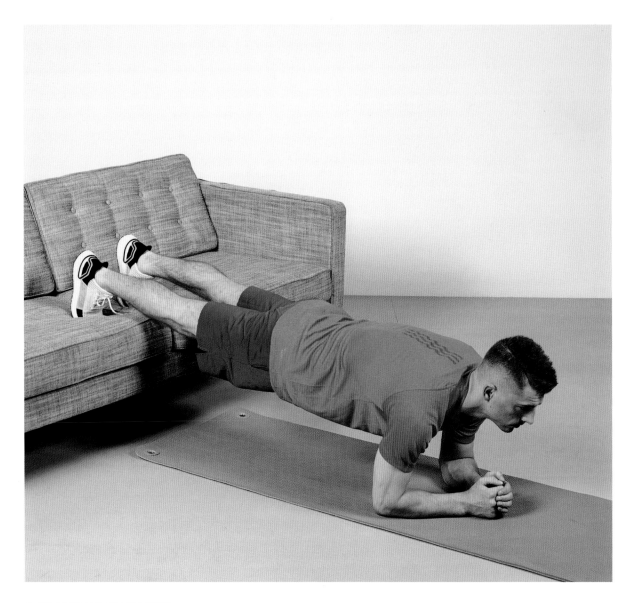

3. PLANK WITH ELBOWS ON FLOOR

By elevating your feet, you increase the difficulty of the plank.

Ensuring that your elbows are directly under your shoulders and that you're up on your toes, hold a plank position with your feet elevated on the sofa.

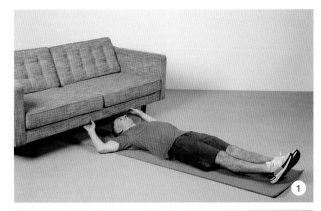

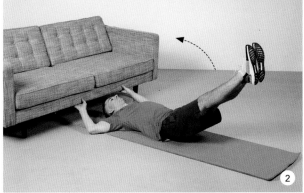

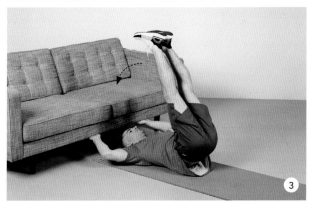

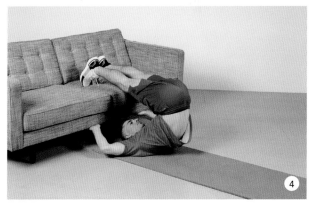

4. LEG LIFTS WITH HANDS UNDERNEATH SOFA

This works your lower abs as well as building lower back mobility.

Lie on your back facing away from the sofa, with straight legs and your hands under the sofa.

Keeping your legs straight, raise them off the floor, pressing your lower back into the floor.

Once your legs pass 90 degrees, release your lower back and, as your legs continue over your head for a toe touch on the sofa, allow it to peel fully off the floor.

Return to the start position with control and repeat.

5. PRESS-UP CLIMBS

A dynamic planking movement that's a workout for your upper body too.

Set-up in a press-up hold position with your hands on the edge of the sofa.

Step one hand down to the floor.

Follow with the other hand and then climb back up to the start position.

Keep working in this way, alternating your hands.

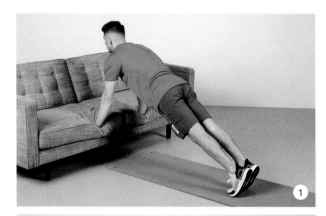

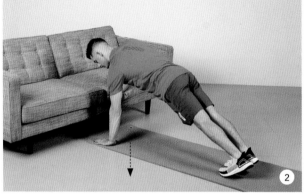

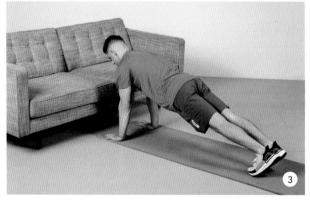

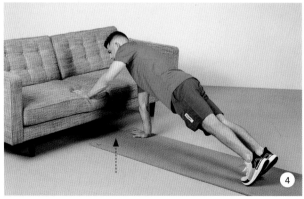

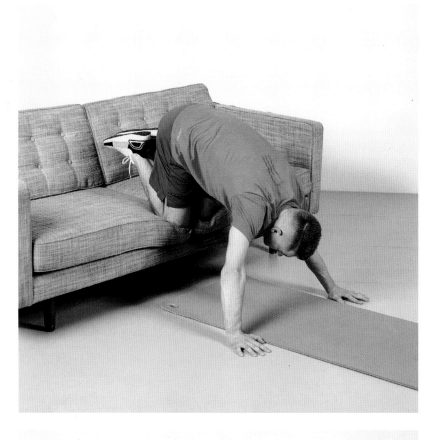

6. HANDSTAND DIPS WITH KNEES ON SOFA

The press-up type movement throws the emphasis onto your upper chest and shoulders.

Kneel on the edge of the sofa and place your hands, slightly more than shoulder width apart, on the floor about a foot from the sofa.

Pivoting on your knees, lower your head towards the floor by bending your arms. You should aim for a 90-degree bend in your arms with your upper arms parallel to the floor.

Lift by straightening, not locking, your arms and repeat.

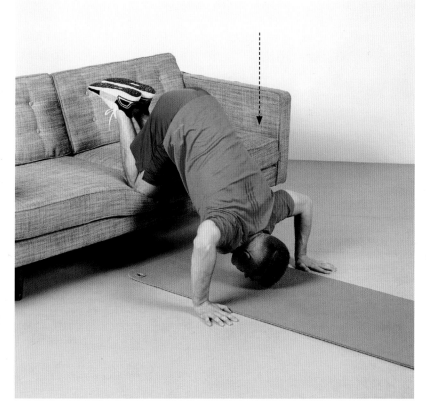

OUCH! WHY AM I SORE?

Don't be surprised or alarmed if your muscles feel sore 24–72 hours after a workout – especially if it contains new exercises, you haven't trained for a while or you've increased the number of cycles. Known as DOMS (Delayed Onset Muscle Soreness), it's thought to be caused by the tiny micro tears and traumas that training results in. Although this might sound dramatic, these tears and the body repairing them is how your muscles get stronger and adapt to exercise. Next time you repeat the workout, you'll probably find that you suffer far less soreness, or even none at all.

Following my recovery tips, including a good cool-down and stretch, will help to reduce muscle soreness and, if it's your legs that are sore, a light walk or spin on a bike can also help. Making sure that you build up your training progressively and don't suddenly ramp things up is the best prevention, though. However, a bit of soreness is no bad thing and shows that you've given your body a good workout.

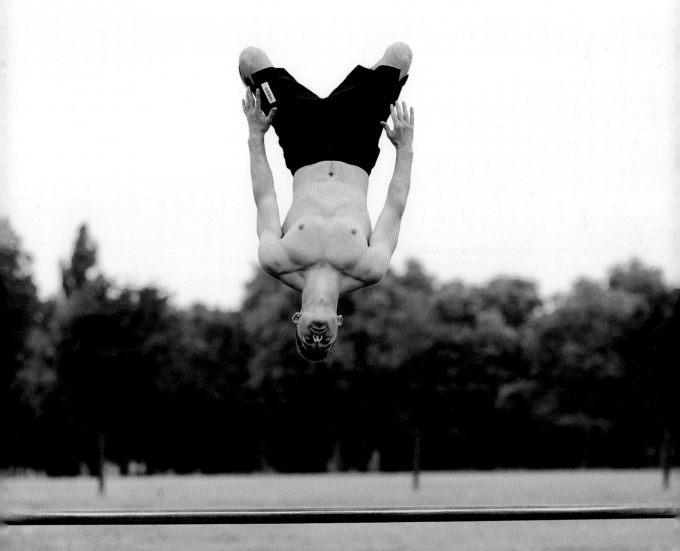

CUSHION CRUSHER WORKOUTS

4 MINUTES PER CYCLE
2–4 CYCLES
30 SECONDS EACH EXERCISE
10 SECONDS REST BETWEEN EXERCISES
1 MINUTE REST BETWEEN CYCLES

The Cushion Crusher Workouts are a great complement to the Sofa Workouts and, by alternating them, you'll keep your body guessing, get brilliant all-over workouts and prevent boredom. Kit is truly minimal: all you need is a cushion or a pillow.

The timings are the same as the Sofa Workouts, making them just as time-efficient and easy to fit into your schedule.

CUSHION CRUSHER WORKOUT – LEVEL 1

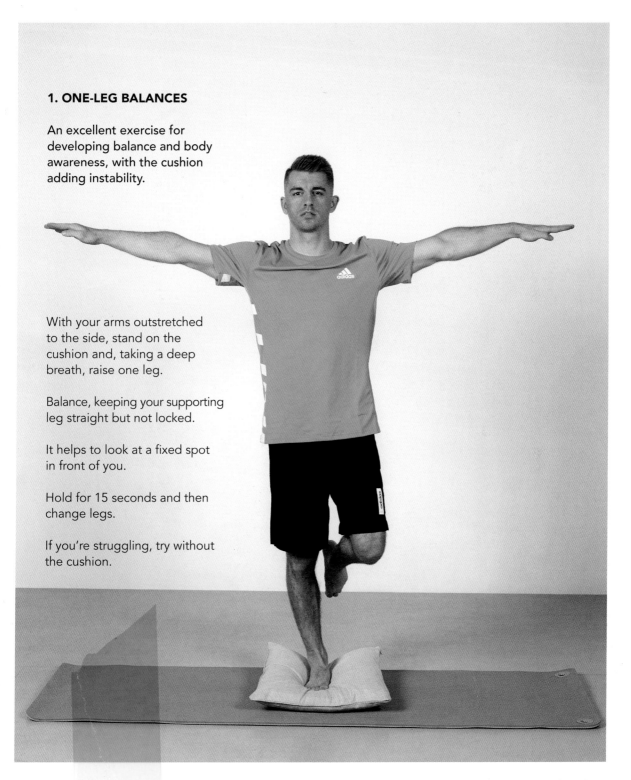

1. ONE-LEG BALANCES

An excellent exercise for developing balance and body awareness, with the cushion adding instability.

With your arms outstretched to the side, stand on the cushion and, taking a deep breath, raise one leg.

Balance, keeping your supporting leg straight but not locked.

It helps to look at a fixed spot in front of you.

Hold for 15 seconds and then change legs.

If you're struggling, try without the cushion.

2. LEG TOUCHES

This works on trunk strength and also hamstring flexibility.

Sit on the floor with your legs straight out in front of you and toes pointed.

Hold the cushion out in front of you at shoulder height.

Holding your trunk stable and without leaning back, raise one leg towards the cushion. Don't worry if you can't quite reach it, just go to the point where you feel a slight stretch on the back of your leg.

Lower the leg with control, replicate the movement with your other leg and keep alternating.

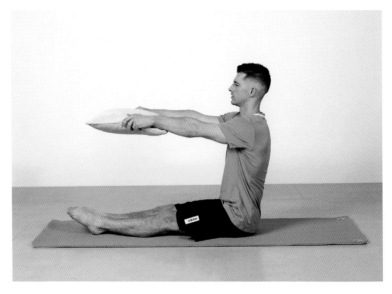

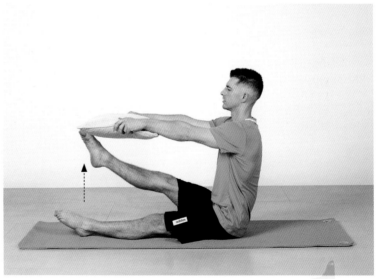

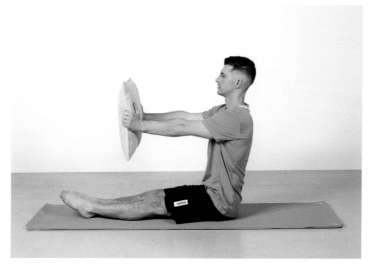

3. CUSHION TWISTS

Hitting your obliques on the sides of your torso and increasing rotational mobility.

Sit on the floor with your legs straight out in front of you and toes pointed.

Hold the cushion out in front of you at shoulder height.

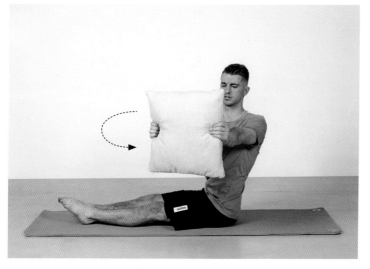

Twist fully to one side from your waist, don't just turn your shoulders.

Return to centre, pause briefly and twist the other way.

Keep alternating.

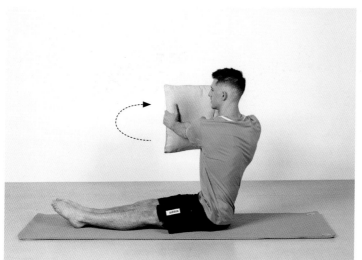

4. DISH HOLD

A static hold that targets your abs.

Lie on the floor with your arms out to the side at 45 degrees and legs elevated and bent at 90 degrees.

Balance the cushion on your shins.

Contract your abs and lift your arms, head, shoulders and upper back off the ground.

Hold this position by maintaining tension in your abs.

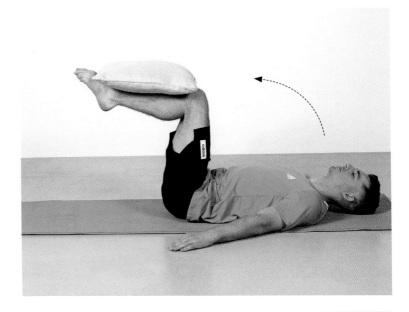

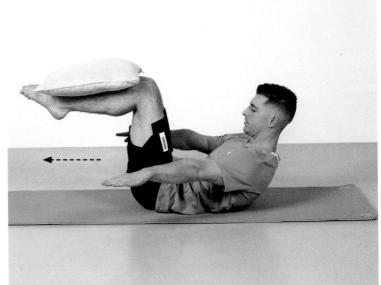

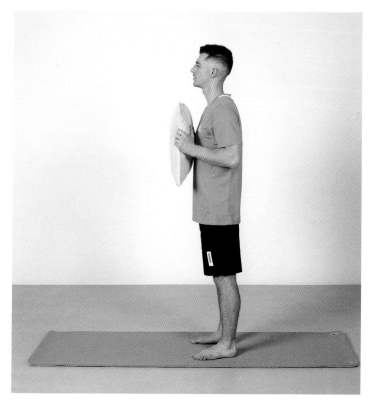

5. AIR PRESS-UPS

This might look easy but, by the end of 30 seconds, I guarantee the front of your shoulders will be burning.

Stand with your feet hip width apart and hold the cushion in both hands at chest height.

Without leaning backwards or forwards, push the cushion away from you by straightening your arms.

Bring the cushion back to your chest and repeat the movement.

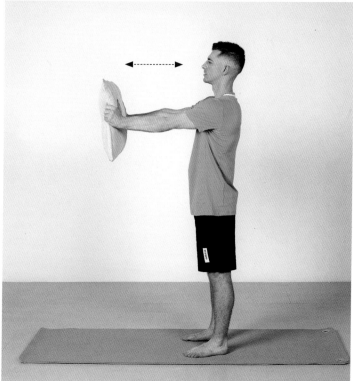

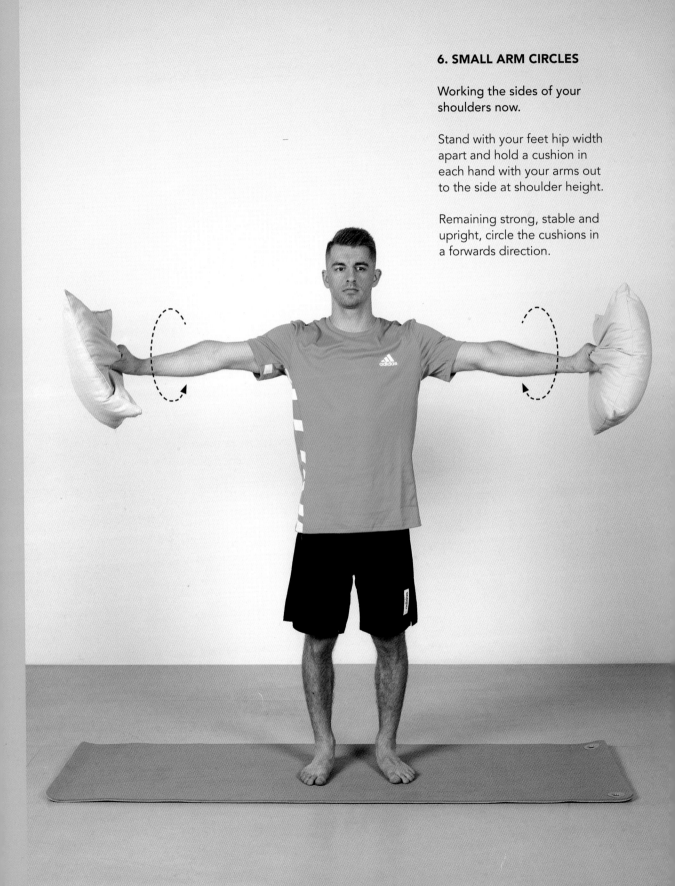

6. SMALL ARM CIRCLES

Working the sides of your shoulders now.

Stand with your feet hip width apart and hold a cushion in each hand with your arms out to the side at shoulder height.

Remaining strong, stable and upright, circle the cushions in a forwards direction.

CUSHION CRUSHER WORKOUT – LEVEL 2

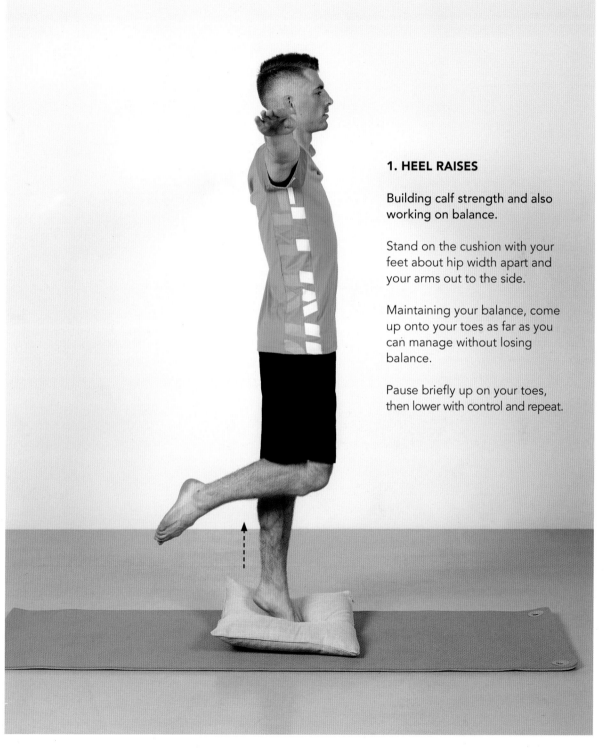

1. HEEL RAISES

Building calf strength and also working on balance.

Stand on the cushion with your feet about hip width apart and your arms out to the side.

Maintaining your balance, come up onto your toes as far as you can manage without losing balance.

Pause briefly up on your toes, then lower with control and repeat.

2. SQUAT HOLD

With a focus on leg strength and balance, this is a great exercise for preparing for more advanced squat-type movements.

Stand on the cushion with your feet about hip width apart and your arms out in front.

Leading with your backside, squat down as low as you feel you can manage. As a minimum, this should be with your legs bent at a 45-degree angle but the ideal is a 90-degree angle, your thighs parallel to the floor.

Hold this position.

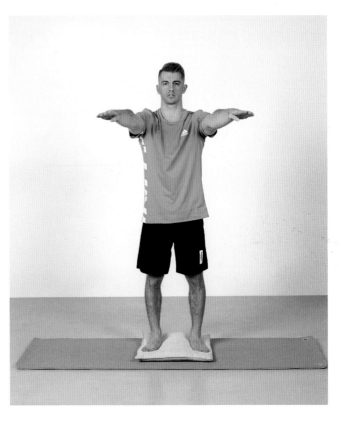

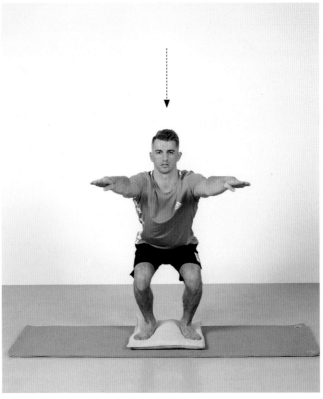

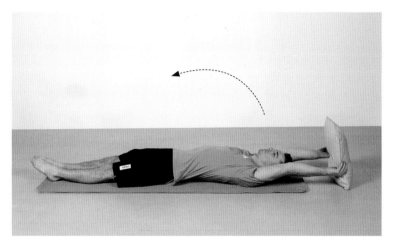

3. SIT-UPS WITH STRAIGHT LEGS

A tough variant on regular sit-ups.

Lie on your back on the floor, with your legs straight.

Hold your cushion with both hands and, keeping your arms straight, take it back over your head and touch the floor behind you.

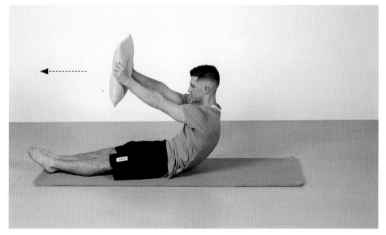

Bring your arms forwards again and, as the cushion comes over your head, sit up. Try to use your abs and not momentum.

Lower with control and repeat.

If you find this movement too hard on your lower back, bend your knees and only come partially up.

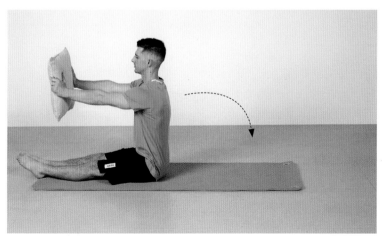

4. TUCK LEG CUSHION TWIST LYING ON BACK

Building on the Cushion Twists (page 67), this movement takes oblique conditioning and lower back mobility to the next level.

Lie on your back with your legs together, bent at 90 degrees and elevated.

Hold the cushion with both hands, arms vertical and straight.

Contract your abs to lift your torso slightly off the floor.

Maintaining ab tension, simultaneously twist your upper body and the cushion one way and the legs the other. Both sides should come close to the floor but not actually touch.

Come back to centre, work the other way, and keep alternating.

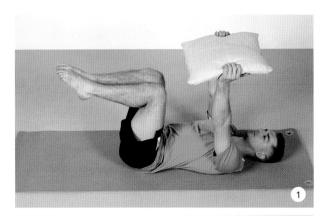

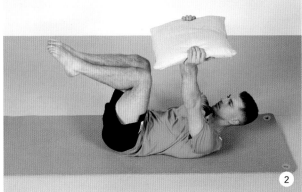

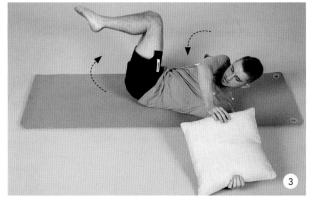

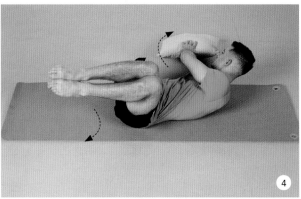

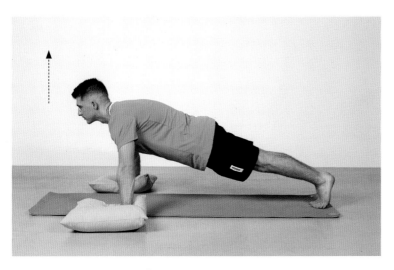

5. WIDE-ARM PRESS-UPS ON CUSHIONS

Press-ups are a classic upper body conditioner but work your core hard too. The wide hand position here emphasises the chest and the cushions add instability, further increasing the difficulty.

Adopt a press-up position with hands wider than shoulder width apart and on your cushions.

Lower your chest by bending your arms, looking to achieve a 90-degree angle with your upper arms parallel to the ground.

Lift by straightening, but not locking, your arms and repeat.

If you find this movement too hard, you can drop your knees to the floor.

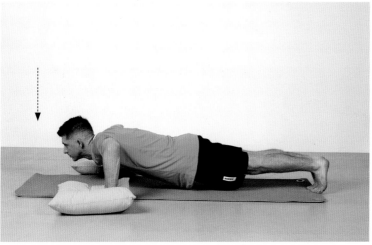

6. ARM LIFTS

Working both your shoulders and core stabilisers, these are surprisingly tough following the press-ups.

Get onto your hands and knees with your hands shoulder width apart on the cushions.

Keeping your head up and looking forwards, alternately raise each cushion to shoulder height.

As you raise and lower, focus on keeping the rest of your body level.

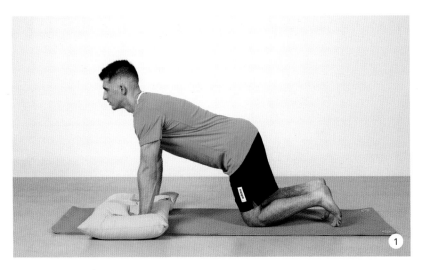

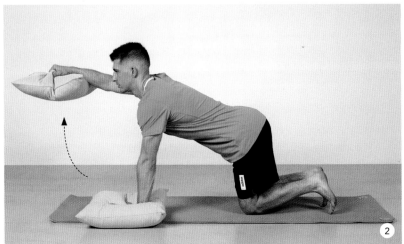

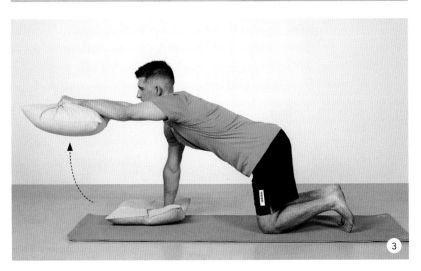

CUSHION CRUSHER WORKOUT – LEVEL 3

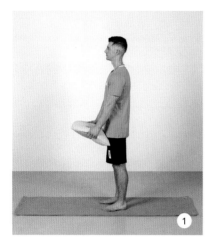

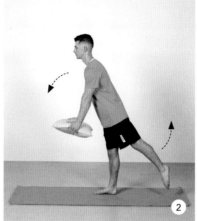

1. ARABESQUE LOWERS

A gymnastic staple and a true test of balance, strength, control and stability.

Stand upright with your feet close together and hold a cushion with both hands straight out in front of you.

By hinging forwards with your upper body and raising one leg straight behind you, lower your cushion towards the ground. As with all balance exercises, keep your head up and try to focus on a fixed point.

Try to keep your standing leg straight and try to create as straight a line as possible from your raised leg to your head and shoulders.

Lower with control, switch legs and continue to alternate.

2. SQUAT HOLD HEEL RAISES

Combining the Heel Raises
(page 71) and Squat Holds
(page 72) for Level 2, this is an
excellent lower body workout.

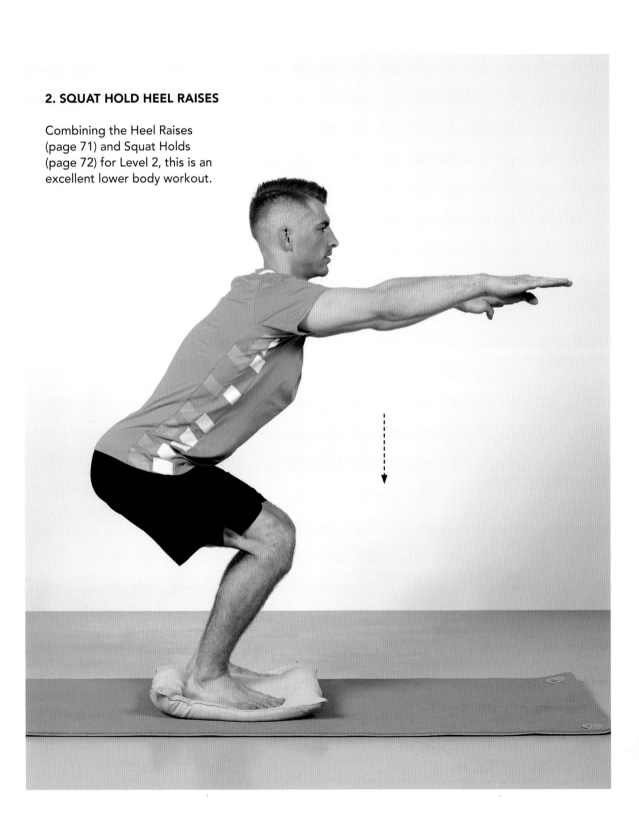

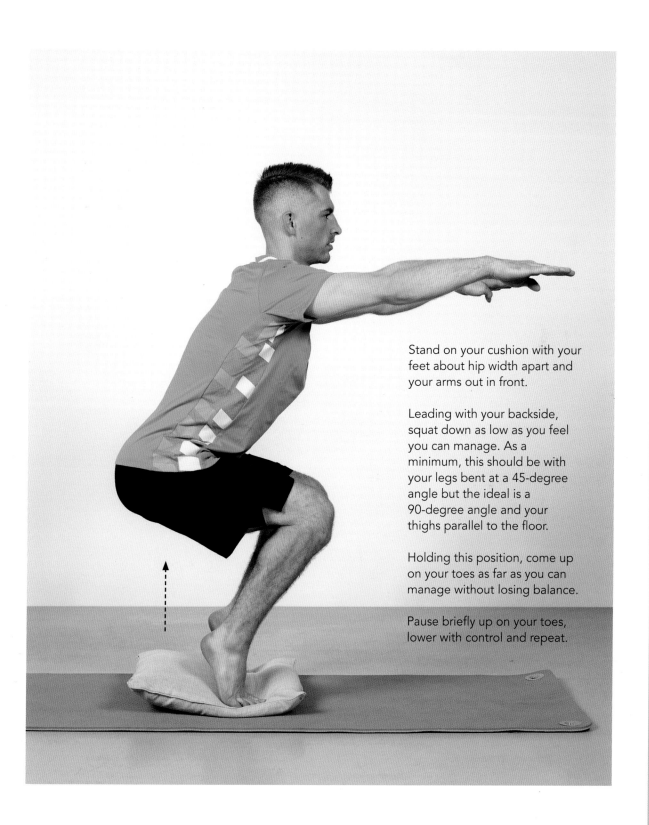

Stand on your cushion with your feet about hip width apart and your arms out in front.

Leading with your backside, squat down as low as you feel you can manage. As a minimum, this should be with your legs bent at a 45-degree angle but the ideal is a 90-degree angle and your thighs parallel to the floor.

Holding this position, come up on your toes as far as you can manage without losing balance.

Pause briefly up on your toes, lower with control and repeat.

3. LEG LOWERS

A powerful exercise for strengthening your lower abs and developing hamstring flexibility.

Lie on your back with your hands behind your head, legs straight and your cushion held between your feet.

Push your lower back into the ground and, trying to maintain this pressure and contact, lift your legs to a 90-degree angle or as far as your hamstring flexibility allows.

Lower with control but not fully back to the ground and repeat.

If you struggle to maintain lower back contact with the ground or struggle with hamstring flexibility, you can have a slight bend in your legs.

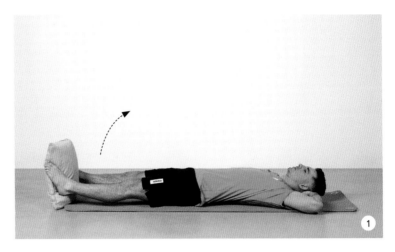

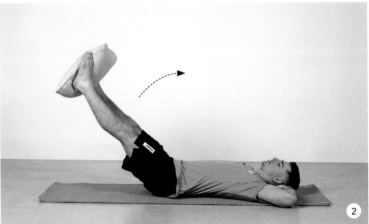

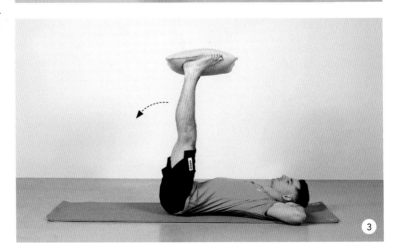

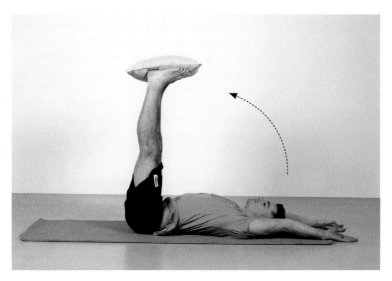

4. HALF V-SITS

Moving straight on from the Leg Lowers (opposite), this switches the emphasis to your upper abs.

Start in the top position of the Leg Lowers, with your legs straight at 90 degrees and a cushion between your feet. Again, if your hamstrings are tight, you can have a bend in your legs.

Have your hands on the floor above your head.

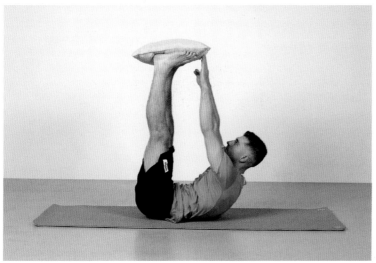

Raise your arms off the floor and forwards and, as they pass over your head, contract your abs to lift your torso off the ground and aim to touch your cushion with your fingertips.

Return with control to the start position and repeat.

5. FRONT SUPPORT WALK

A dynamic planking movement that will work your upper body and core.

Adopt a narrow grip press-up position with your hands just in front of your cushion.

Lift and move one hand out to a wide position.

With the other hand, lightly tap close to the leading hand and then return it back to its starting position. Return the leading hand to its starting position.

As soon as your hands are back to the start position, work out to the other side and continue cycling through.

Aim to be as fluid as possible, minimising pauses but maintaining control.

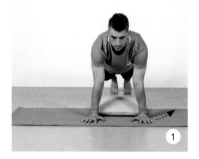
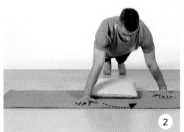
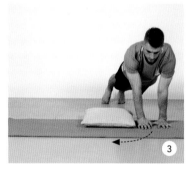
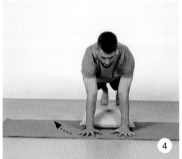
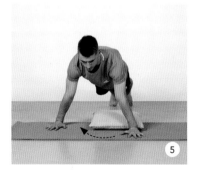
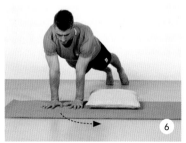

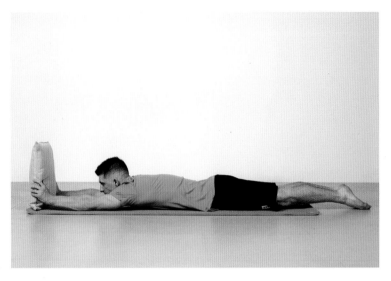

6. UPPER LIFTS

You've worked your abs hard so this exercise for your lower back helps to balance things out.

Lie face down, looking forwards and with your cushion held out in front of you with straight arms.

Focusing on your lower back and backside, lift your cushion, arms and chest off the floor.

Pause in the top position, lower and repeat.

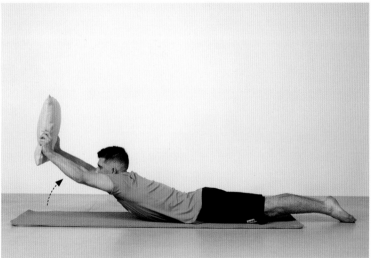

YOU CAN'T SPOT REDUCE

We've all got bits of our body that we don't like and that, no matter what we do, seem to stubbornly cling on to fat. A common myth is that by working a particular area hard, such as doing loads of sit-ups for your stomach or dips for the backs of your arms, you can get rid of the fat in that area. Unfortunately, this just isn't true and, although you'll develop the muscle group you're targeting by focusing on it, you won't cause any preferential fat burning in that area. This is why all of my workouts focus on your whole body and don't specify hips, bums or tums. By working all of your major muscle groups regularly and consistently and with a balanced and healthy diet, you'll see your body composition change and those troublesome areas will start to shape up.

Another common misconception is that muscle will turn to fat if you stop exercising. This is simply untrue as muscle and fat are anatomically different tissue types. If you stop exercising and therefore stop stimulating a muscle, it can reduce in size or atrophy. At the same time, if you fail to reduce your calorie intake to compensate for not training, you'll gain some fat. But one doesn't turn into the other.

Finally, electronic gadgets that claim to 'tone muscles' aren't going to give you a six-pack or perfectly sculpted arms. These devices were originally developed for rehabilitation and to prevent muscle loss after injury or in bed-bound patients. They're effective in this role but simply don't provide enough training load to stimulate growth and they're definitely not going to have any impact on any fat overlying the muscle.

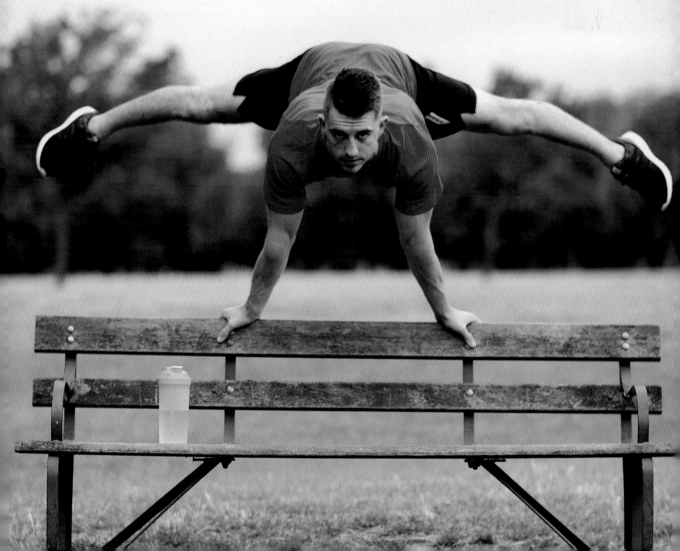

TOTAL BODY WORKOUTS

AIM FOR 2–4 CYCLES
4 MINUTES PER CYCLE
30 SECONDS EACH EXERCISE
10 SECONDS REST BETWEEN EXERCISES
1 MINUTE REST BETWEEN CYCLES

With the excellent levels of strength and mobility that you will have developed from the Sofa Workouts, you can now progress to these Total Body Workouts.

Utilising the same structure and timings and requiring no kit, they'll feel familiar but will definitely take your conditioning to another level. You'll notice that many of the movements are more gymnastic in feel and build on the great foundations that you've already laid down.

TOTAL BODY WORKOUT – LEVEL 1

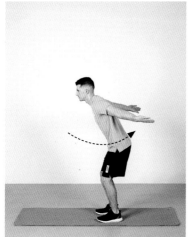
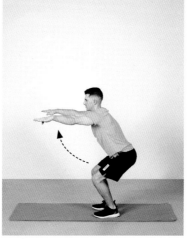

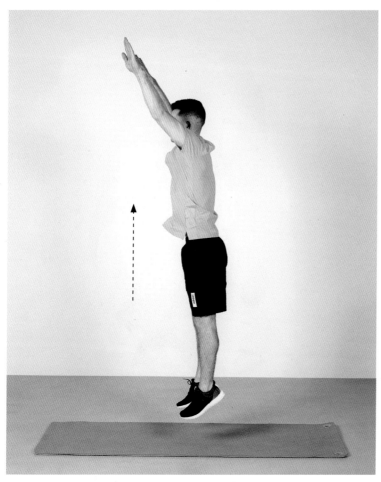

1. STRAIGHT JUMPS TO STICK

The 'stick' in this exercise refers to a gymnastic landing. It focuses primarily on explosive strength but will also challenge your balance and co-ordination, and will definitely raise your heart rate.

Stand with your feet hip width apart.

Swing your arms back and, as you do so, sink into a ¾ squat.

Swing your arms forwards to shoulder height and use this momentum to explode upwards.

In the air, tap your feet together and return to hip width.

Absorb your landing with soft knees and repeat.

2. 3 HOPS

More balance work, but you'll also be working your cardiovascular system and targeting your calves.

With arms out to the side to aid balance, come up onto the ball of one foot and hop rapidly 3 times.

On the third hop, land on your other foot and keep alternating.

Your hopping leg is straight but keep your ankle and knee soft.

You should be looking for speed, not height: imagine you're standing on a hot surface.

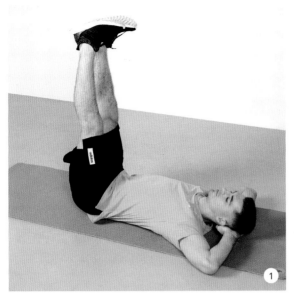

3. SINGLE LEG WINDSCREEN WIPERS

Focusing on core strength but also developing hamstring, hip and lower back mobility.

Lie on your back with hands behind your head and both legs straight and elevated to as close to 90 degrees as you can manage.

Brace your core and try to push your lower back into the floor.

With control, lower one leg out to the side.

When you've almost reached the floor, return the leg to the start position and repeat with the other leg.

Continue to alternate legs.

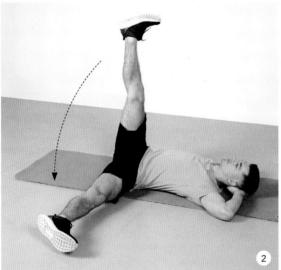

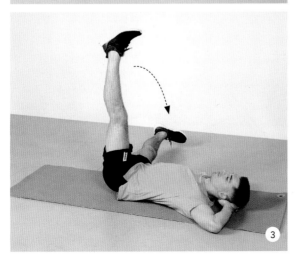

4. FRONT SUPPORT

This should be a familiar exercise to you and is a go-to for core strength.

Hold the 'up position' of a press-up.

Maintain a straight line from your shoulders to heels, no sagging or arching.

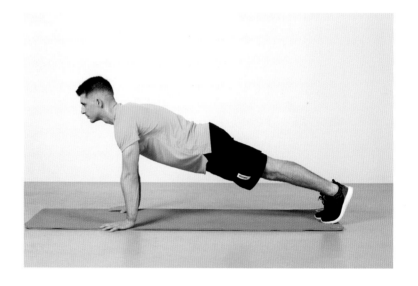

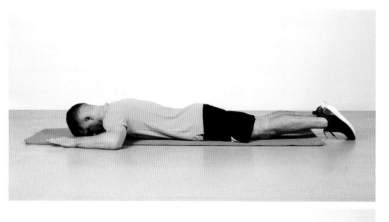

5. HEAD ON FLOOR SHOULDER LIFTS

Focusing on shoulder and chest mobility and upper back strength. Although this might feel like a bit of a recovery exercise, it's brilliant for counteracting the hunched posture that desk work can cause.

Lie face down on the floor with your forehead on the ground and arms bent at 90 degrees.

Lift your arms off the floor by pulling your shoulder blades together.

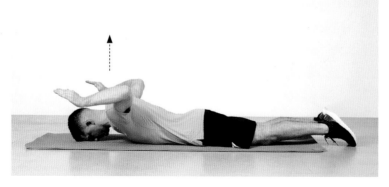

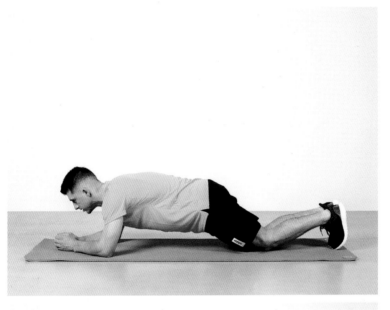

6. FOREARM PRESS-UPS

Although this will hit your upper body, it's also effectively a plank-type exercise, so your core will be working hard too.

Adopt a stretched-out forearm plank position, with your knees down. Unlike a regular plank, you don't want your elbows directly under your shoulders but in front of them.

Raise your body and lift your forearms off the floor by straightening your arms.

Lower and repeat.

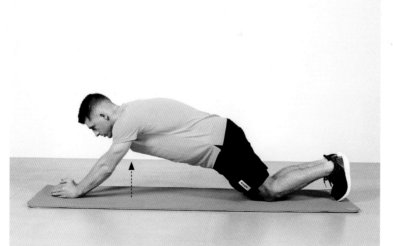

TOTAL BODY WORKOUT – LEVEL 2

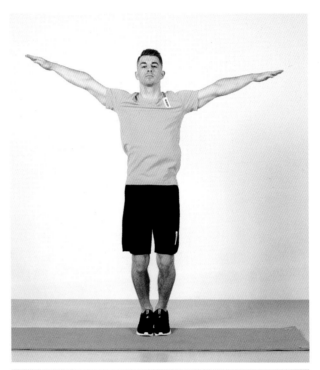

1. SMALL REBOUND JUMPS

An extension of the warm-up that'll raise your heart rate but will also develop rebound speed and calf muscle endurance.

Stand with your arms out to the side, slightly above shoulder height; imagine you've just finished a gold medal-winning routine!

Come up onto the balls of your feet and, keeping knees and ankles soft, begin to jump.

Focus on speed and fast rebound, rather than height; how many can you do?

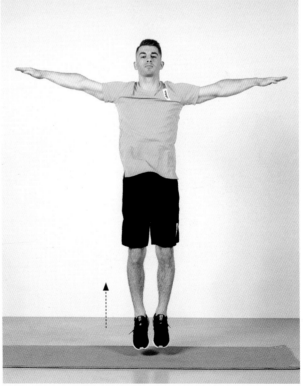

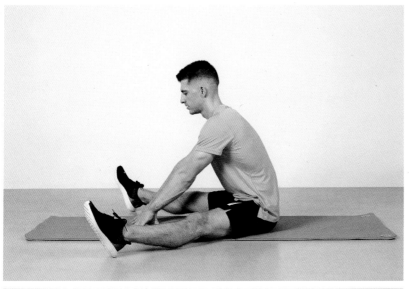

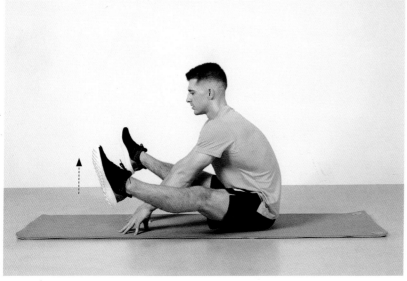

2. SITTING STRADDLE LEG LIFTS

Challenging lower abdominal and hip strength and hamstring flexibility.

Sit on the floor, hinging slightly forwards from your waist, with your legs straight and out to the side and your fingertips touching the ground in front of you.

Lift both legs off the ground, aiming to keep them straight and your toes pointed.

Lower with control and repeat.

3. DISH ROCKS

Probably one of the toughest but most effective core strengtheners you can do.

Lie on your back and, with your hands extended over your head, elevate your legs and upper torso off the ground.

Hold this position and, maintaining control, rock forwards and backwards.

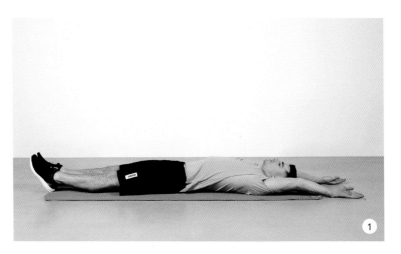

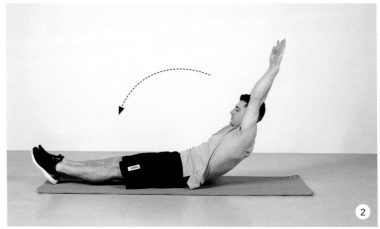

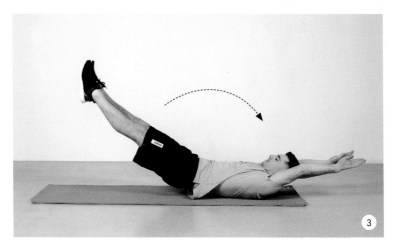

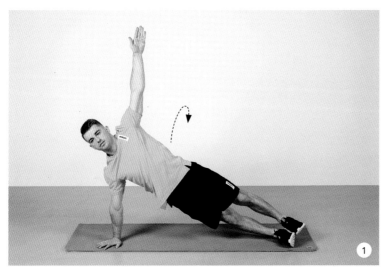

4. SIDE PLANK TRANSFERS

An advanced progression of the side plank that, along with working your obliques, will also really test your shoulder strength and mobility.

Start in a side plank position.

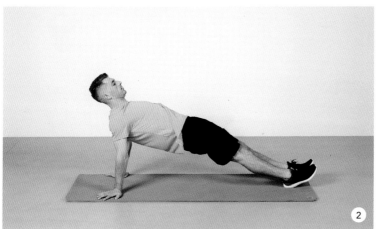

Once you feel balanced, rotate backwards, bringing your hand to the floor and your body into a back bridge position.

Carry on the rotation to bring you into a side plank on the other side.

Pause briefly, reverse the movement and continue to alternate.

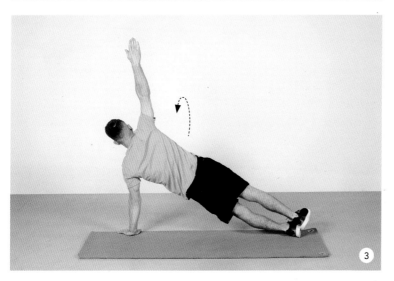

5. FRONT SUPPORT SHOULDER SHRUGS

Working the muscles of your upper back and a static hold for your core.

Adopt the 'up position' of a press-up.

Keeping your arms straight, allow your torso to drop by bringing your shoulder blades together.

Lift by spreading your shoulder blades and repeat.

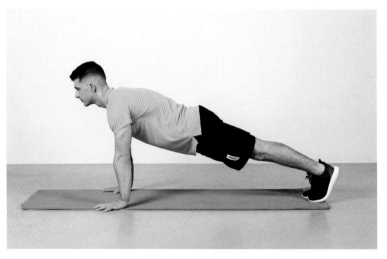

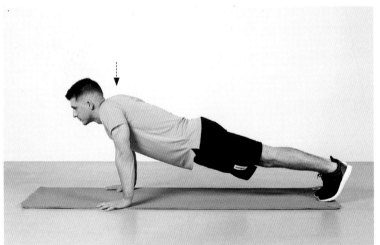

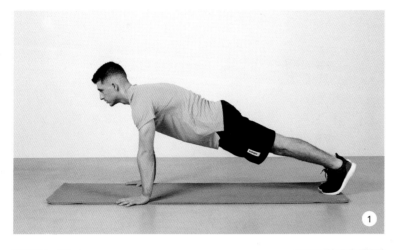

6. SQUAT-ON PREP

Raising your heart rate at the end of the workout and building lower body strength and muscular endurance.

Adopt the 'up position' of a press-up.

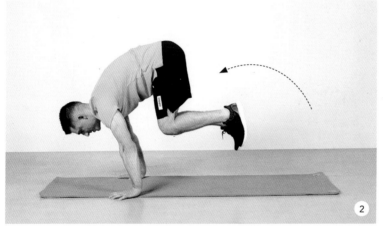

Jump your legs forwards, bringing your knees between your arms and aiming for your feet to come to just behind your hands.

Jump your legs back to the start position and repeat.

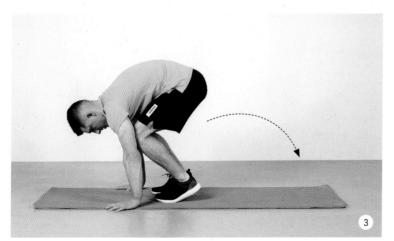

TOTAL BODY WORKOUT – LEVEL 3

1. JUMP HALF TURN TO STICK

A progression from the Level 1 movement (page 87), which requires more explosion and balance on the landing.

Stand with your feet hip width apart.

Swing your arms back and, as you do so, sink into a ¾ squat.

Swing your arms forwards to shoulder height and use this momentum to explode upwards.

In the air, perform a 180-degree turn and, along with soft knees on the landing, brace to prevent further rotation.

Repeat, working in the same direction for half the time and then work the other way.

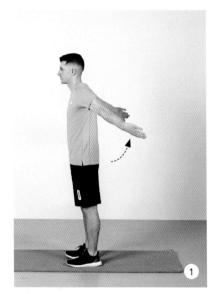
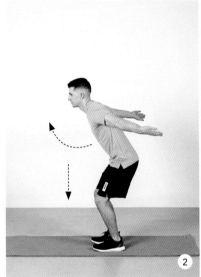
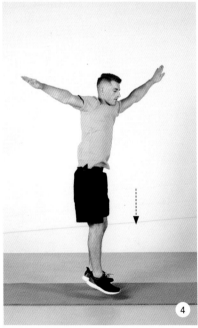
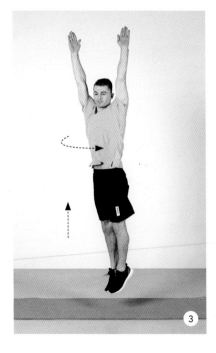

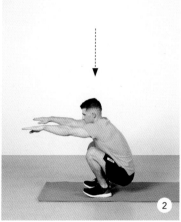

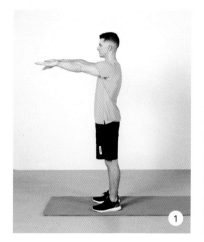

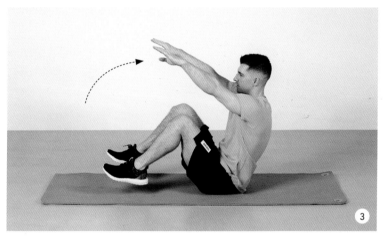

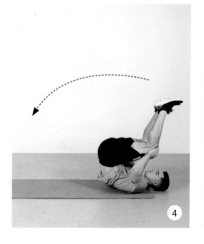

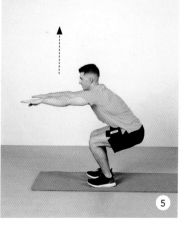

2. ROLL BACKS

Effectively an advanced-level sit-up that demands excellent levels of core strength and mobility.

Stand with feet slightly narrower than hip width apart and hands out in front of you.

With control, sink into a deep squat; it should only be in the final 15–30cm before your backside hits the floor that you should start to fall back.

Bring your hands to your knees and, as you roll back onto your upper back and shoulders, bring your knees to your ears.

As you roll forwards, throw your hands forwards and use the momentum you generate and a strong abdominal contraction to bring you back up onto your feet.

Come up to a ¾ squat and repeat.

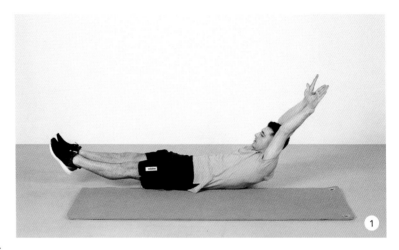

3. DISH TO ARCH

Bringing a dynamic component to a dish that forces you to shift the emphasis alternately from your abs to your lower back.

Lie on your back and, with your arms extended overhead, elevate your legs and torso off the ground into a dish.

Keeping tension, roll onto your side and, as you transition onto your front, ensure that your chest and legs are elevated off the floor in an arch.

Roll again in the same direction and back into a dish.

Return in the opposite direction and keep alternating in this way.

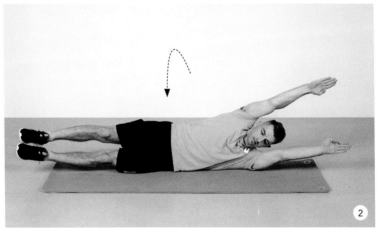

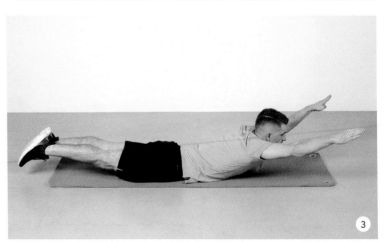

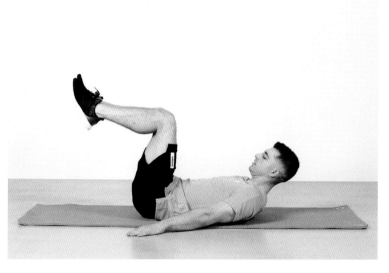

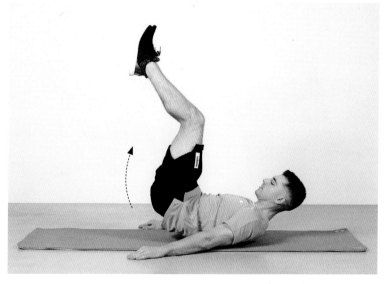

4. BUM LIFTS WITH TUCKED LEGS

With your stomach muscles already fatigued, this exercise really focuses in on your lower abs.

Lie on your back with your arms out at 45 degrees to your body, head off the floor and legs elevated to 90 degrees and slightly bent.

By contracting your abs, lift your backside and lower torso off the ground.

Lower with control and repeat.

5. WRIST PRESSES

Forearm strength is often neglected. With this exercise, you're working your core too.

Adopt the 'up position' of a press-up.

Keeping your arms straight, lift your palms off the ground and come up onto your fingers.

Lower and repeat.

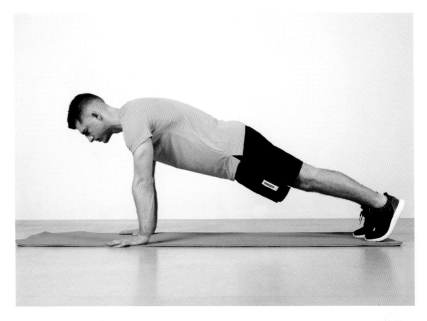

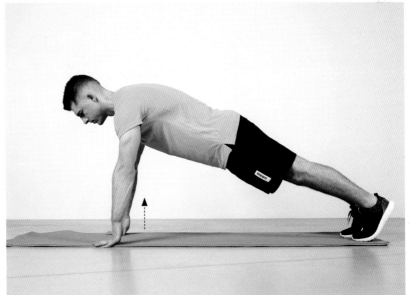

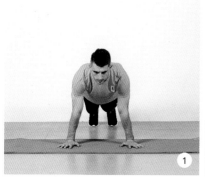

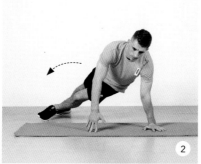

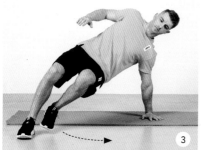

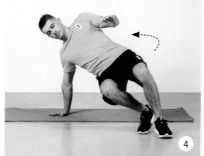

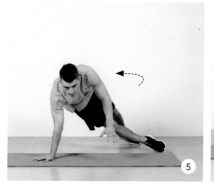

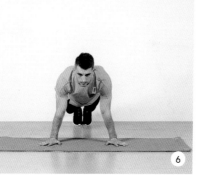

6. CIRCLES

A whole body movement, developing strength, mobility and body awareness.

Adopt the 'up position' of a press-up.

Maintaining as much body extension as you can, walk your feet round, shifting onto one hand, through a side plank and into a back bridge.

Carry on round, through a side plank on the other side and back to the start position.

Repeat in the opposite direction and keep alternating.

MAX'S LIFE: *MOTIVATION*

I guess I'm lucky in that I don't get those days when I don't want to get up and go to the gym to train very often. I think that's mainly because I love what I do and, even after all the hours I've spent in the gym training, it still fires me up. One thing that always helps to keep me motivated, though, is thinking of that long-term goal. For me, it might be my next major championships or the Olympics and knowing that every quality workout I do will contribute towards me performing at my best. For you, it might be being healthier, looking good for your summer holiday or being fitter for your 5-a-side league.

Once you've got that long-term goal, put in place a number of tangible and controllable short-term goals that will be stepping stones towards this. These could be managing a certain number of reps of an exercise, doing three exercise sessions a week or even drinking enough water. Avoid goals that you don't have so much control over, such as weight loss targets, as these often result in disappointment and demotivation.

I'd strongly recommend you to ditch your scales as, whether it's hydration level or changes in body composition, there are so many factors that govern your weight that you can't control. It's not unusual, when people start exercising, for them to put on some weight as they gain some muscle and increase their blood volume. It's far better and more motivating to gauge your progress by your workout performance.

You'll find with my workouts that, because of their structure and the type of exercises, you'll see progress almost from session to session. This might be being able to squeeze out a few more reps or, because you've become more agile and coordinated, just managing one full rep of a challenging movement. It'll all be moving you forwards and you can draw motivation from that.

A while ago, I was trying to encourage my parents to exercise more and, although it was an uphill battle to start with, once they got going, got into it and started to see the benefits, they went from strength to strength and now regular exercise is just part of their lives. It can be tough to start with and you might have days when you really don't feel like doing it but try to push through and establish that habit.

A good tip, if you are having a low motivation day, is to make a deal with yourself that, as long as you start a workout, if, once you've done, say, the warm-up or one cycle through and it's still not happening, you can quit guilt free. I guarantee, 99 per cent of the time, once you've got started, you'll see it through. Also, get yourself a workout buddy; training is so much more fun and easier with someone else.

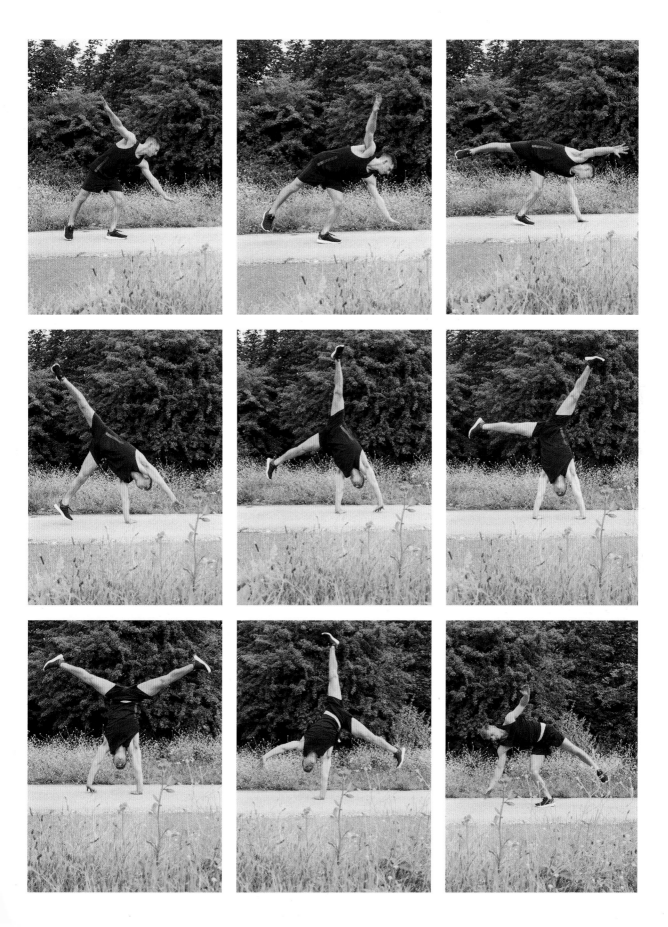

HOME BAR WORKOUTS

2–3 MINUTES PER CYCLE
1–5 CYCLES
30 SECONDS EACH EXERCISE
10–30 SECONDS REST BETWEEN EXERCISES
90 SECONDS REST BETWEEN CYCLES

A pull-up bar is a great piece of workout kit and, as you'll see from these workouts, can be used for so much more than just pull-ups.

Many gyms will have suitable pull-up bars, as will park gyms and, if you have a suitable beam or wall, are fairly cheap and easy to install at home. The cheapest at-home option are doorway bars and, although you may have to modify some of the exercises to accommodate their lower height, they can still be really effective.

The exercises in these workouts are extremely demanding and Level 3 especially is a 'Pro Level' workout. You should be proficient at my Level 3 Total Body Workouts (page 98) before attempting the Level 1 Home Bar Workout.

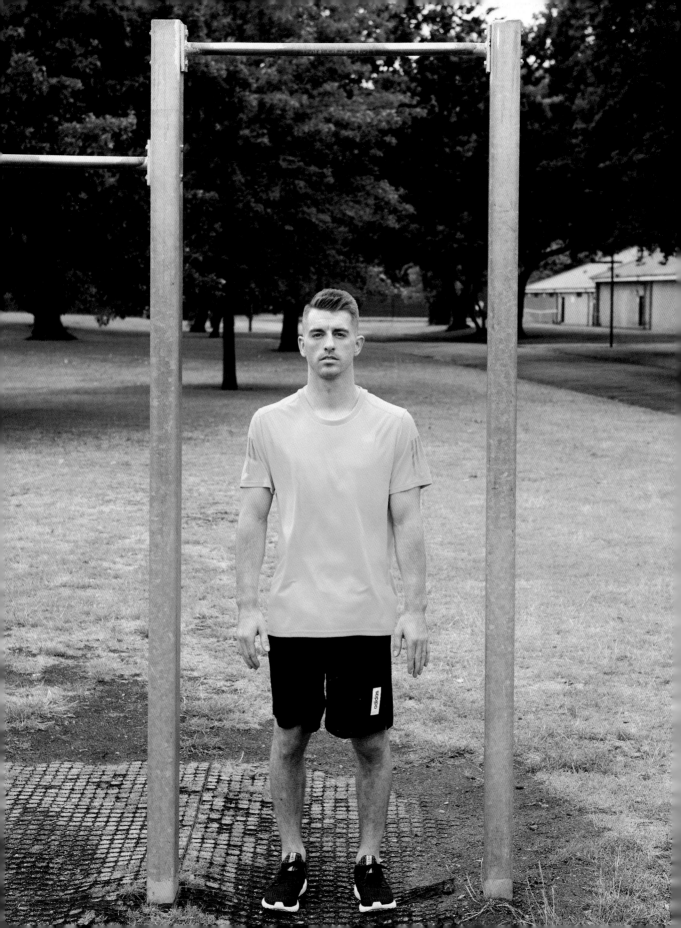

STRUCTURE

The structure of both the Home Bar Workouts and Rings Workouts differ from my previous workouts and reflect their advanced nature.

Still devote 5–10 minutes following my 5-minute Pre-workout Warm-up Routine (see page 28) before your session and do at least my 5-minute Post-workout Stretch Routine (see page 36) afterwards.

There are 3 exercises per cycle.

Aim to work for 30 seconds per exercise. You will probably find that you might struggle to keep going for the full 30 seconds and, given the exercises, this shouldn't be a surprise. Simply do as many reps as you can manage in good form and either just hang for the remaining time or take some extra rest.

Don't rush into the next exercise, take 10–30 seconds to recover.

Take a 90-second rest between cycles.

The first time you try the workout, just do 1–2 cycles and, as you become familiar with it, try to build up to 5 cycles.

Once you can manage 5 cycles at Level 1, move to Level 2 but drop back down to 1–2 cycles before building up again. Do the same when you step up to Level 3.

HOME BAR WORKOUT – LEVEL 1

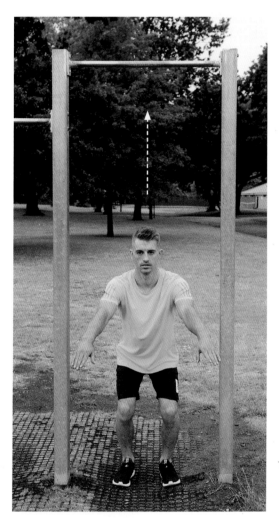 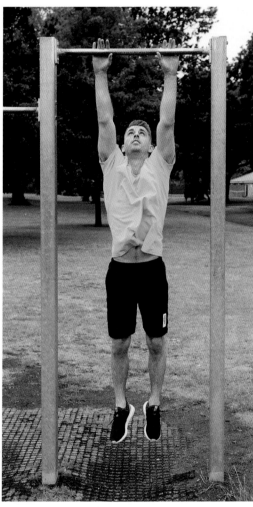

1. SQUAT JUMP TO TOUCH BAR

An explosive movement that will develop leg strength and power and will also ramp up your heart rate.

Stand under the bar with your feet about hip width apart.

Sink into a squat, keeping your head up, arms out in front and bringing your thighs parallel to the floor.

Explode upwards to touch the bar or higher.

Land with soft knees, sinking into the squat to absorb the impact before exploding upwards again.

2. HANGING CRUNCHES

This exercise combines a dead hang for your grip and general upper body strength and a leg raise to hit your lower abs.

Hang with your palms facing forward and a slightly wider than shoulder width grip.

Minimising any swinging, bring your knees up to your chest.

Lower with control, aiming for a 90-degree bend in your legs as they pass hip level.

Continue to lower until legs are fully straight, or as straight as your bar height allows, and repeat.

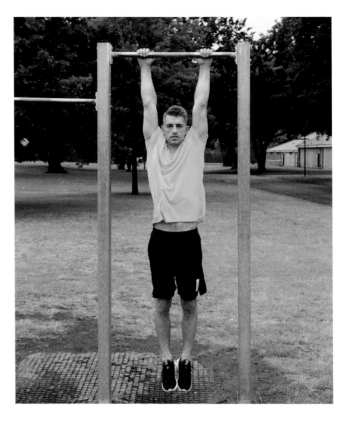

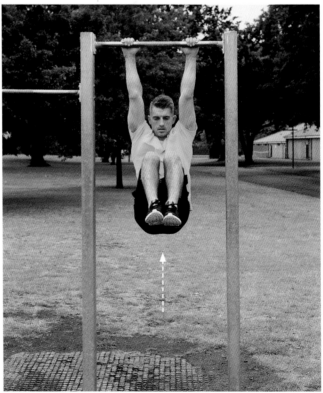

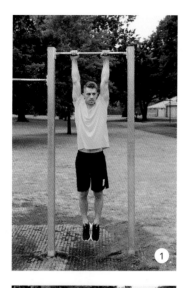

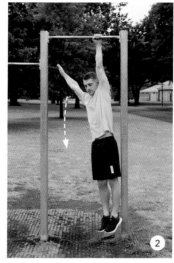

3. MONKEY SWINGS

A really challenging exercise that'll build grip and overall upper body strength but will also test your trunk stability.

Hang with your palms facing forwards and a shoulder width grip.

Minimising any swinging, remove one hand from the bar and circle it backwards in a controlled manner to return it to the bar.

Repeat with the other hand and continue to alternate.

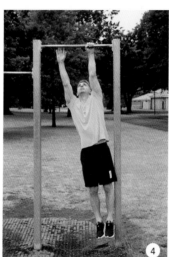

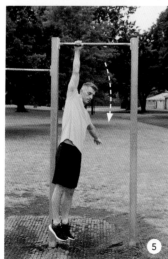

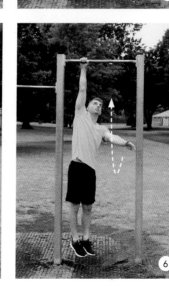

HOME BAR WORKOUT – LEVEL 2

1. SCISSOR LUNGES TO TOUCH BAR

Building on from the squat jumps, this adds the instability of a lunge set-up and is a real test of balance and explosive strength.

To set up, stand slightly behind the bar with your feet hip width apart. Take a step forwards and slightly to the side and drop down into a lunge position. You're looking for your front thigh to be parallel to the floor, your back knee to be almost touching the floor and both legs bent to 90 degrees.

Explode upwards from this position to touch the bar and, as you do so, switch your legs around in the air.

Land with soft knees, and sink into the lunge to absorb the impact before exploding upwards again.

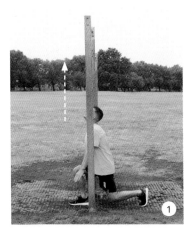

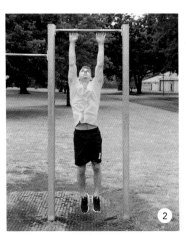

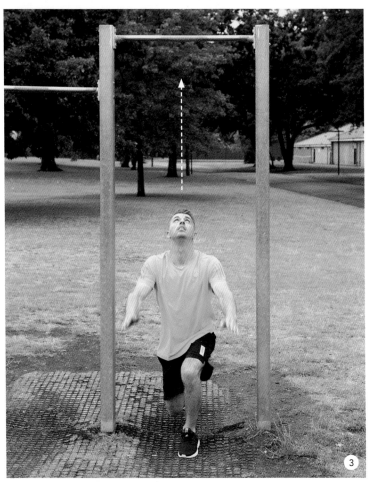

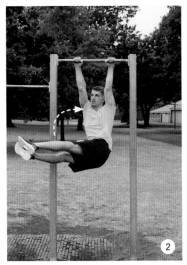

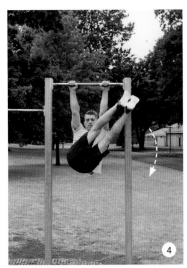

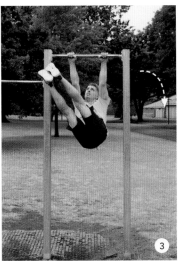

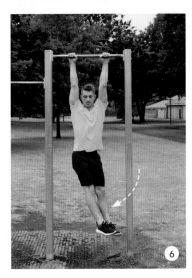

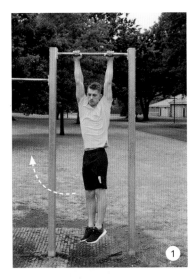

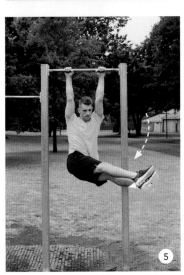

2. LEG LIFT CIRCLES

This progression from the Hanging Crunches (page 110) provides a real test of abdominal strength and control.

Hang with your palms facing forwards and a slightly wider than shoulder width grip.

Minimising any swinging throughout the movement, keep your legs straight and, with a slight twist of your torso, lift them up and to the side.

Continue the circle of your legs, aiming to bring your toes past your hands and then down the other side and to the start position.

Repeat in the other direction and continue to alternate.

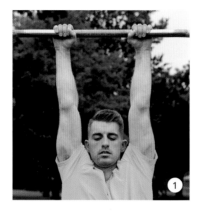

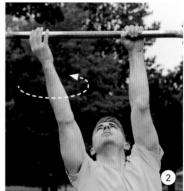

3. GRASP CHANGES

Another hang movement that, by switching your grip, constantly changes the muscle focus.

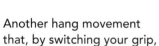

Hang with your palms facing forwards and a shoulder width grip.

Controlling any swinging, remove one hand from the bar and, without allowing your body to drop, switch to an underhand, palm facing back, grip.

Follow with the other hand.

Continue cycling between over- and underhand grip.

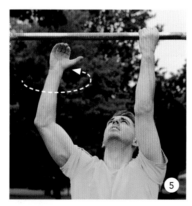

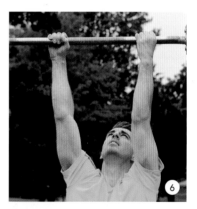

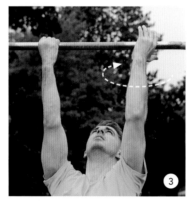

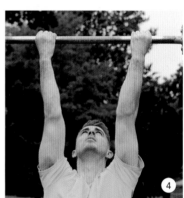

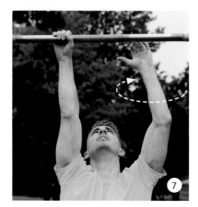

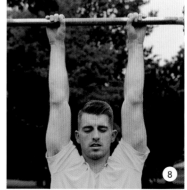

HOME BAR WORKOUT – LEVEL 3

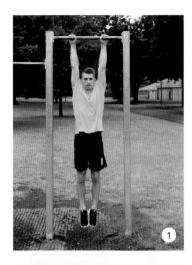

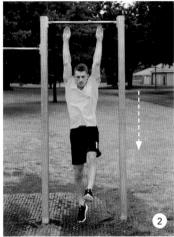

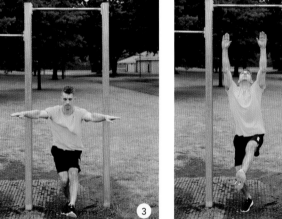

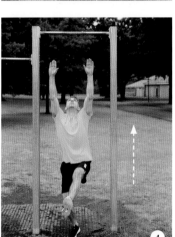

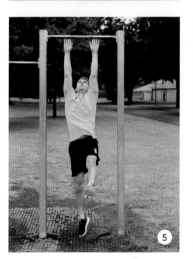

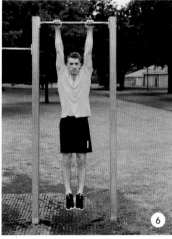

1. ONE LEG SQUAT TO TOUCH BAR

A genuine whole body exercise that requires high levels of strength and balance.

Hang with your palms facing forwards and a shoulder width grip.

Drop from the bar, landing on one leg and absorb the impact by sinking into a single-leg squat.

Explode upwards, catch the bar, switch legs as you hang and repeat.

Keep alternating.

2. ONE-ARM LEG LIFT

An extremely challenging leg lift variant.

Hang with your palms facing forwards and a shoulder width grip.

Let go of the bar with one hand and, avoiding swinging, half circle your legs up on that side to the bar. Try to keep your legs straight.

As you lower with control, return your hand to the bar and, once back in the start position, repeat on the other side.

Keep alternating.

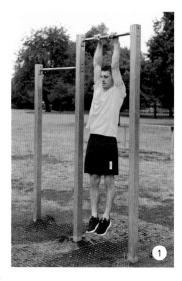

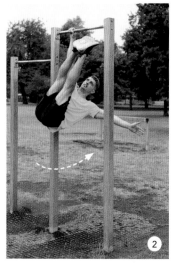

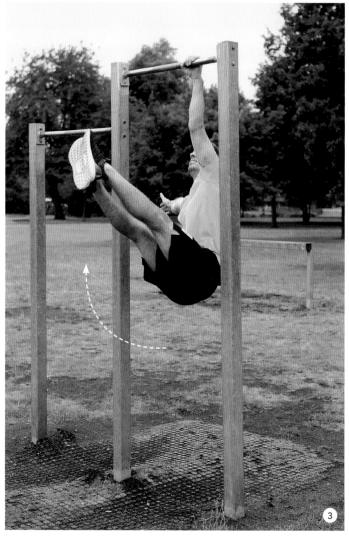

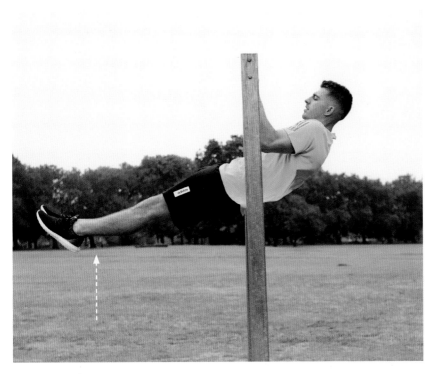

3. POM POMS

A true test of trunk stability, body control and upper body strength. The slower you can do this exercise the better; it's not a swing.

Hang with your palms facing forwards and a slightly wider than shoulder width grip, and pull up so that your eyes are level with the bar.

Keeping tension through your whole body, trying to keep it as straight as possible and with control, lean back and raise your legs.

Aim for as flat a position as you can manage, pause briefly in this position, lower and repeat.

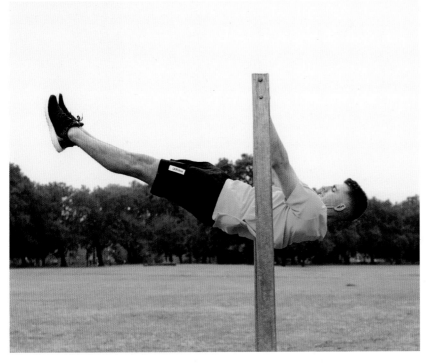

RINGS WORKOUTS

2–3 MINUTES PER CYCLE
1–5 CYCLES
30 SECONDS EACH EXERCISE
10–30 SECONDS REST BETWEEN EXERCISES
90 SECONDS REST BETWEEN CYCLES

Olympic Rings have become very popular and, because of the instability they bring to a number of exercises, can be used to create extremely demanding and effective workouts. They can be hung on a pull-up bar or you can use a suitable beam or joist. Many gyms and CrossFit Boxes have them too.

Follow the same workout structure and progression as described for the Home Bar Workouts (page 106) and, like those workouts, these are advanced sessions so you should have completed Level 3 of the Total Body Workouts (page 98) before attempting them.

RINGS WORKOUT – LEVEL 1

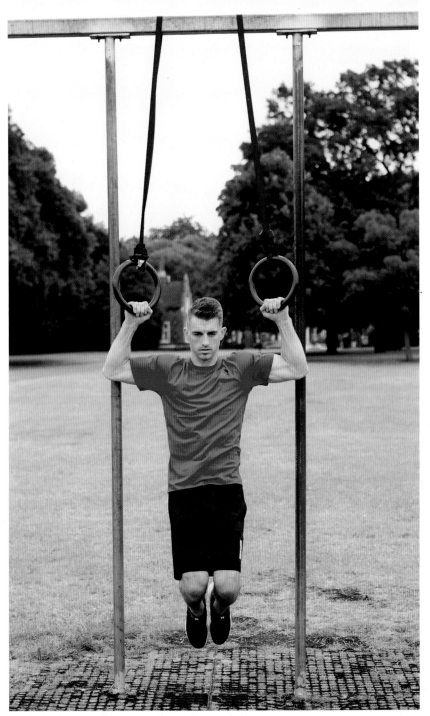

1. CHIN-UP HOLD

This exercise works on upper body strength, especially your biceps, upper back and forearms. Remaining calm and focused in this position is a real physical and mental challenge.

Hang on the rings with your hands facing forwards and, with your legs tucked behind you, pull-up so that your arms are bent at 90 degrees.

Hold this position.

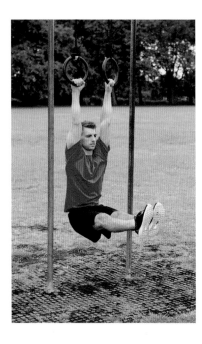

2. HANGING HALF LEVER SCISSORS

The static hang of this exercise continues to target your upper body and then adds in some ab work.

With hands facing forwards, hang at full stretch on the rings.

Keeping your legs straight and avoiding swinging, raise them straight out in front of you. You're looking for your body to form an L shape.

Holding this position, perform controlled scissor kicks.

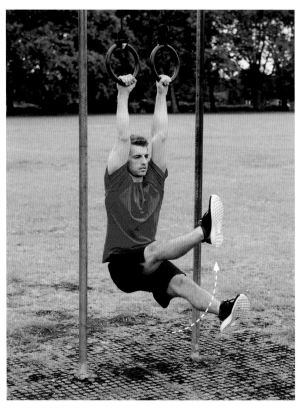

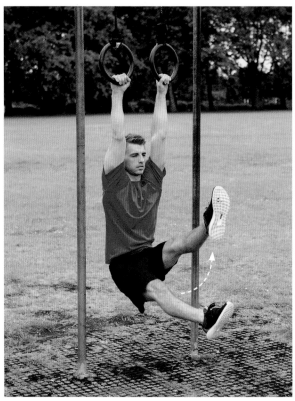

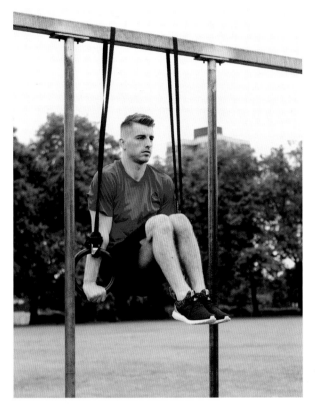

3. RING TURNS IN TUCK

Shifting the hold emphasis onto your chest, shoulders and triceps, the ring turns really work your forearms and, by holding the tuck position, you're also hitting your lower abs.

Push up into a high hold position on the rings and raise your knees to waist height and into a tuck.

Holding this position, rotate the rings so that your palms are facing forwards.

Return your hands to a neutral position and repeat.

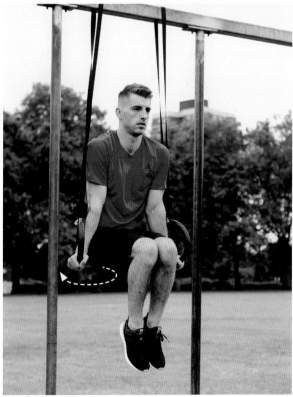

RINGS WORKOUT – LEVEL 2

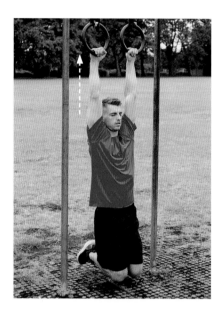

1. WIDE ARM CHIN-UPS

Probably one of the best upper back and biceps exercises you can do.

Hang on the rings with legs tucked underneath you and palms facing forwards.

Pull up and, as you do so, your hands should travel outwards so that, in the top position, the rings are outside your shoulders.

Lower with control and repeat.

It's important not to swing to generate momentum.

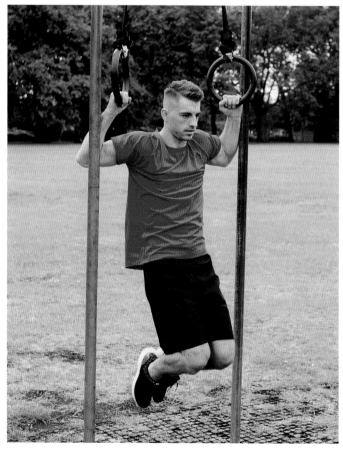

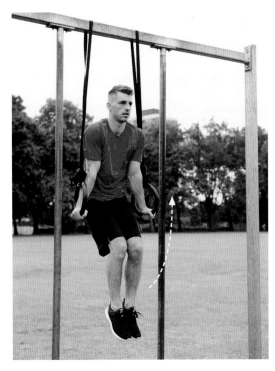

2. TUCK CRUNCHES IN SUPPORT

This focuses on your lower abs but, like all holds, works your upper body hard too.

Push up into a high hold position on the rings.

Bring your knees up to waist height.

Lower with control and repeat.

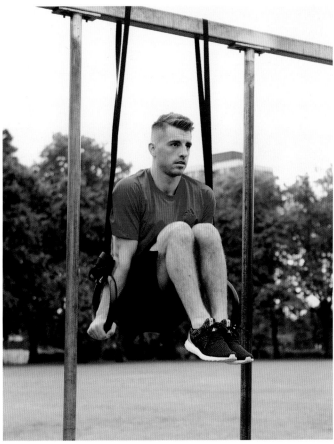

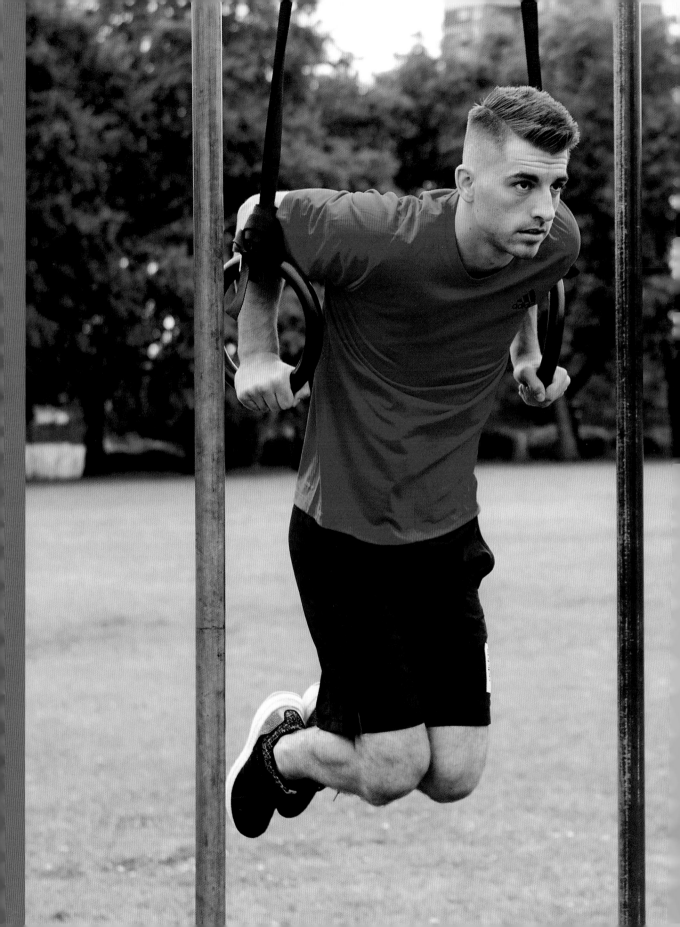

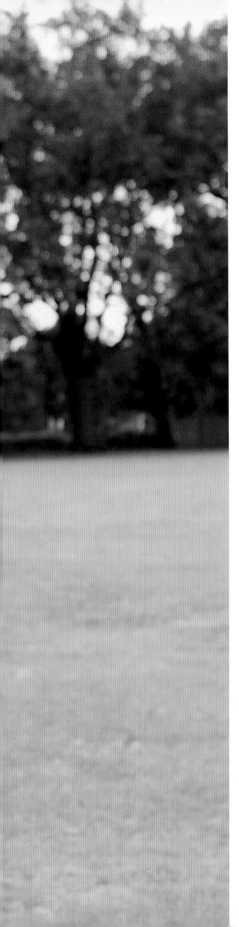

3. DIPS

If the chin-ups were the gold standard for back and biceps, dips will do the same for your chest and triceps.

Push up into a high hold position on the rings.

Leaning forwards slightly, bend your arms and lower into a dip. You can tuck your legs underneath you if you want.

You're looking for your arms to be bent to at least 90 degrees and ideally your shoulders should come level to the rings.

Pause briefly, push back up and repeat.

Avoid 'half reps' where you don't go to full depth. It's better to do 1 or 2 full-range quality reps than a greater number of poor ones.

PERFECT 10 PRO PARK WORKOUTS

10 REPS PER EXERCISE
10 SECONDS BETWEEN EXERCISES
3–5 MINUTES REST BETWEEN CYCLES

Park gyms and fitness trails, with pull-up bars, parallel bars, benches, monkey bars and a whole range of other exercise stations, are brilliant places for building gymnastic fitness. The only thing limiting what you can do is your imagination – and the weather.

Most of my workouts can be adapted to a park gym and, on a sunny day, there's nothing to beat getting out and exercising in the open air.

This Perfect 10 Pro Park Workout is probably the toughest workout in the book and requires excellent levels of all-round fitness. At the very least, you should be proficient at my Level 3 Total Body Workouts (page 98) and ideally should have progressed onto the Home Bar (page 106) and Rings Workouts (page 118) before attempting it.

STRUCTURE

The 10 in the title of this workout refers to 10 exercises, 10 reps and the 10–out–of–10 fitness you'll need to complete it!

Make sure you warm up well, devoting 5–10 minutes to following my 5-minute Pre-workout Warm-up Routine (page 28) before your session. If you've jogged to the park, you can include this as part of your warm-up but still do the mobilisation exercises. At the end, work through my 5-minute Post-workout Stretch Routine (page 36) but you can leave this until you get home if you've run there.

There are 10 exercises in the circuit; work through them in sequence.

Perform 10 reps per exercise, unless specified otherwise in the instructions.

When you first start with this workout, take your time, focus on form and allow as much recovery as you feel you need between exercises.

As you become more familiar with it, slowly build up the pace.

Once you can do one cycle through the 10 exercises, you can build up to 2 or 3 cycles. Take a 3–5 minute rest between cycles.

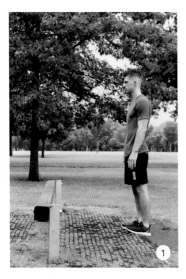

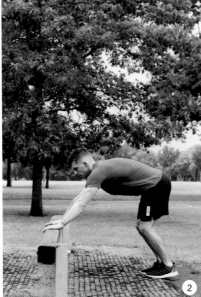

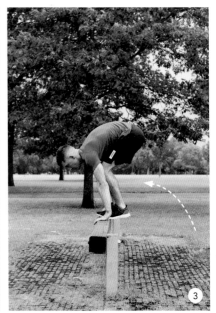

1. SQUAT-ONS

An explosive total body movement that'll get your heart racing and legs burning.

Stand facing a bar or bench, around knee height.

Sinking into a partial squat, lean forwards, bringing your hands to the bar.

Spring up, bringing your feet between your hands and come to a standing position on the bar.

Jump backwards off the bar, land with soft knees to absorb the impact and go straight into the next rep as quickly as possible, minimising contact time with the ground.

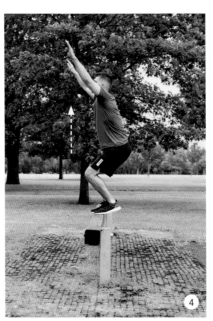

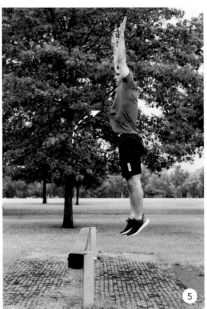

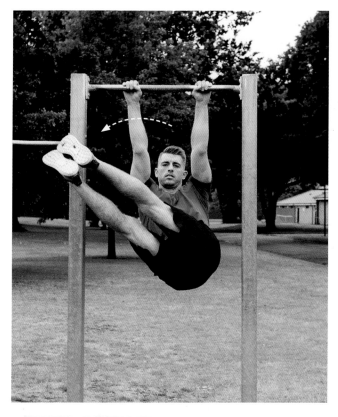

2. WINDSCREEN WIPERS

A dead-hang that works your upper body combined with a killer exercise for your abs.

Hang on a high bar with palms forwards, slightly wider than shoulder width grip.

Raise your legs, keeping them straight, so that your knees are at chest level.

Maintaining body control and balance, 'wipe' your legs from side to side.

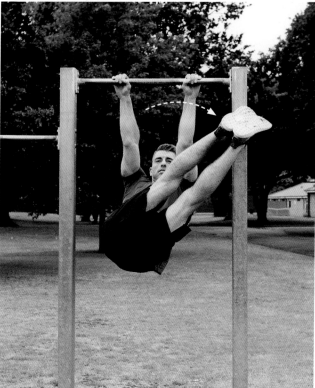

3. UPPER ARMS DIPS

On to the parallel bars for an extremely hard dips variant.

Adopt a support position on the bars with your feet tucked behind you.

Bend your arms and slightly lean forwards to go into a full dip; your shoulders should go below your elbows.

Rock back to bring your upper arms fully onto the bars with your elbows level with your shoulders.

From this position, drop your body lower until your ears are below your elbows but keep your forearms on the bars.

Lift back to elbows and shoulder level.

Repeat and, at the end of the set, press out of the dip to support position.

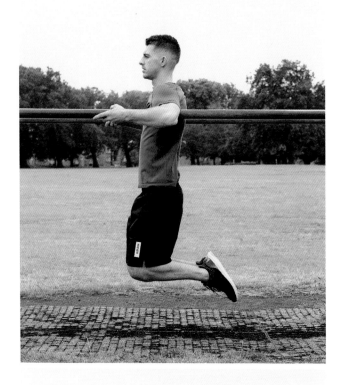

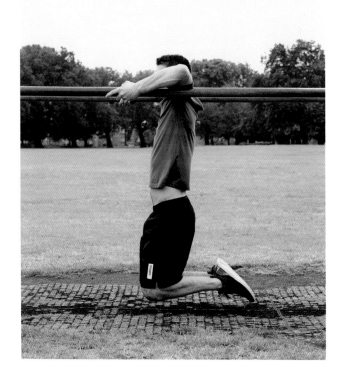

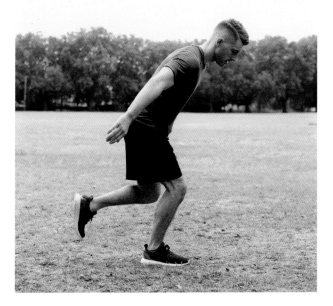

4. ONE LEG HOPPING TUCK JUMPS

A break for your upper body but this is an advanced explosive lower body exercise that'll kick your heart-rate back up.

Stand on one leg, with your hands out to the side for balance, and sink into a partial single-legged squat.

Explode upwards and bring both knees up towards your chest into a tuck.

Land on the same leg you jumped from and, minimising ground contact time, explode up again.

Perform 5 reps on one leg and 5 on the other.

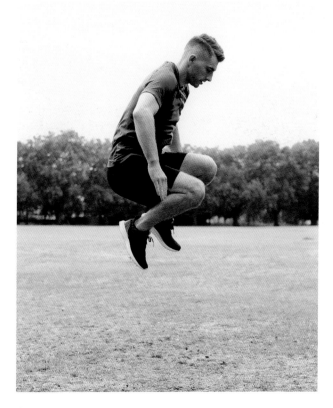

5. LEG LIFTS

Back to the high bar to hit your lower abs.

Hang on a high bar with palms forwards, slightly wider than shoulder width grip.

Keeping your legs straight and minimising swinging, raise them so that your toes come to the bar.

Lower with control and repeat.

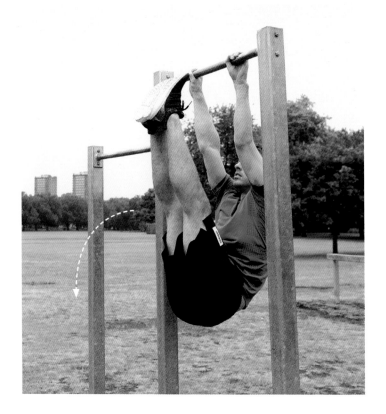

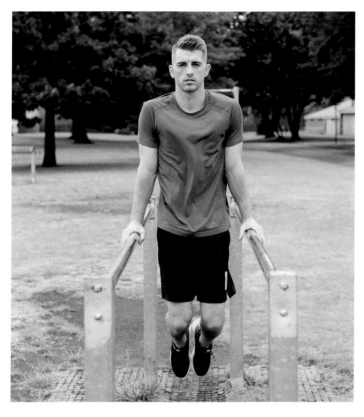

6. DIPS

Standard dips on the parallel bars to target your chest, triceps and shoulders.

Adopt a support position on the bars with your feet tucked behind you.

Bend your arms and slightly lean forwards to go into a full dip; your shoulders should go below your elbows.

Straighten your arms to return to the start position and repeat.

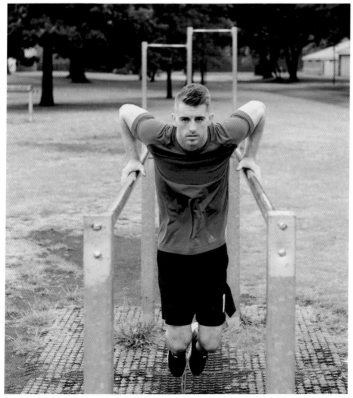

7. TUCK REBOUND JUMPS

These might be slightly easier than the single-legged variant you did earlier in the circuit but, with your legs pre-fatigued, you'll definitely feel them.

Stand with your feet about shoulder width apart.

Partially squat to preload your legs.

Explode upwards and bring your knees to your chest into a tuck.

Extend your legs to land with soft knees and, minimising ground contact time, explode up again.

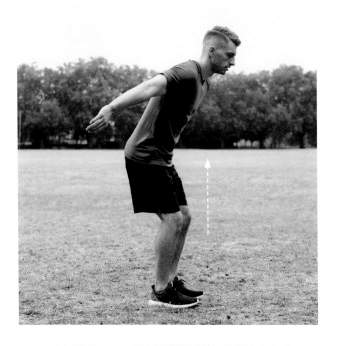

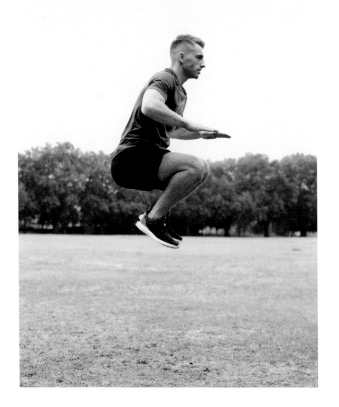

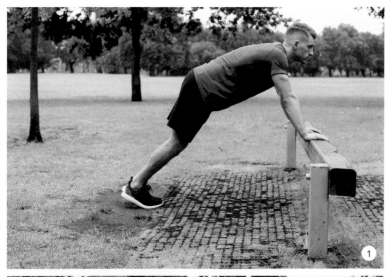

8. TENSION BRIDGE ON BENCH

An advanced plank variant that tests whole body strength and stability.

Start with your hands on the edge of a bench and walk your feet back so that your body is at full extension.

Brace and hold this position for 10 seconds with no arching of your back or sagging of your hips.

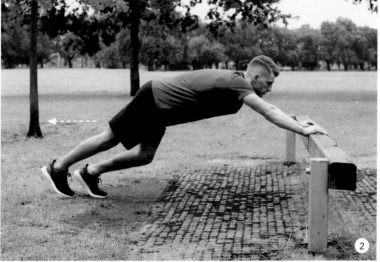

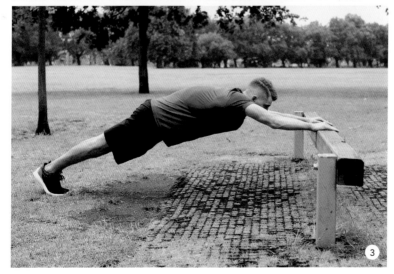

9. SHOULDER SHRUGS IN SUPPORT

Your final visit to the parallel bars to target the muscles of your upper back, neck and shoulders.

Adopt a support position on the bars with your feet pointing straight down.

Keeping your arms straight, lower by shrugging your shoulders up towards your ears.

Lift back up and repeat.

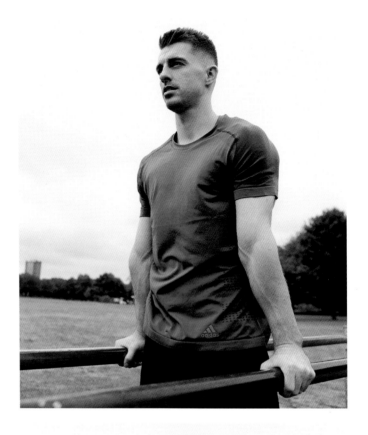

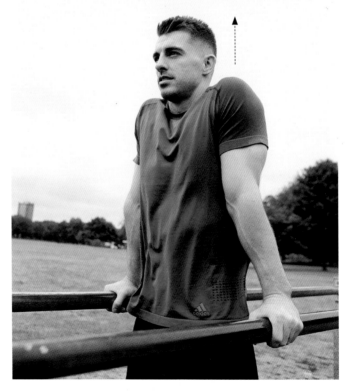

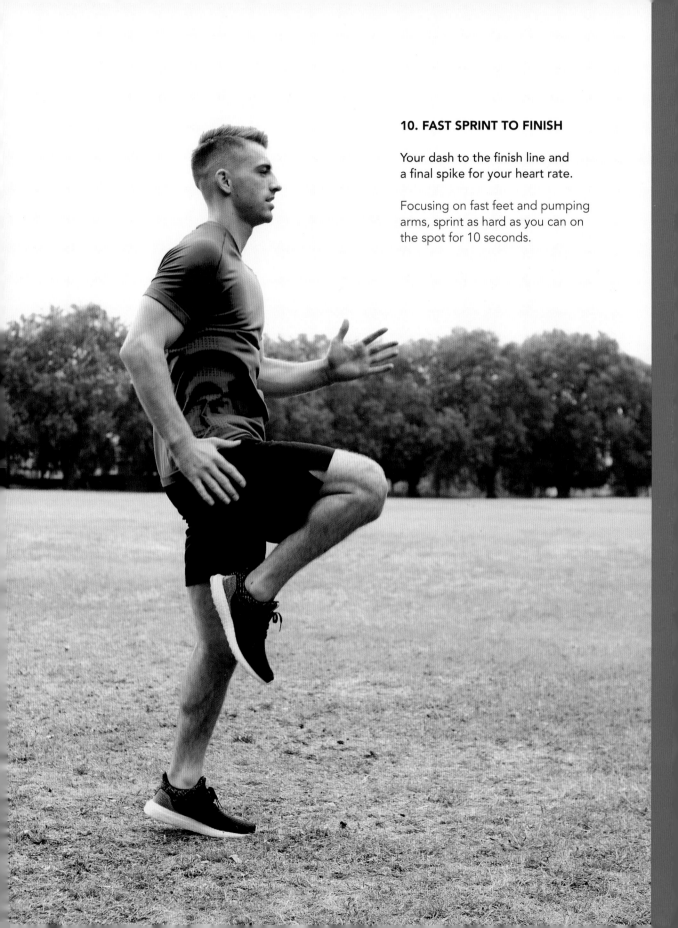

10. FAST SPRINT TO FINISH

Your dash to the finish line and a final spike for your heart rate.

Focusing on fast feet and pumping arms, sprint as hard as you can on the spot for 10 seconds.

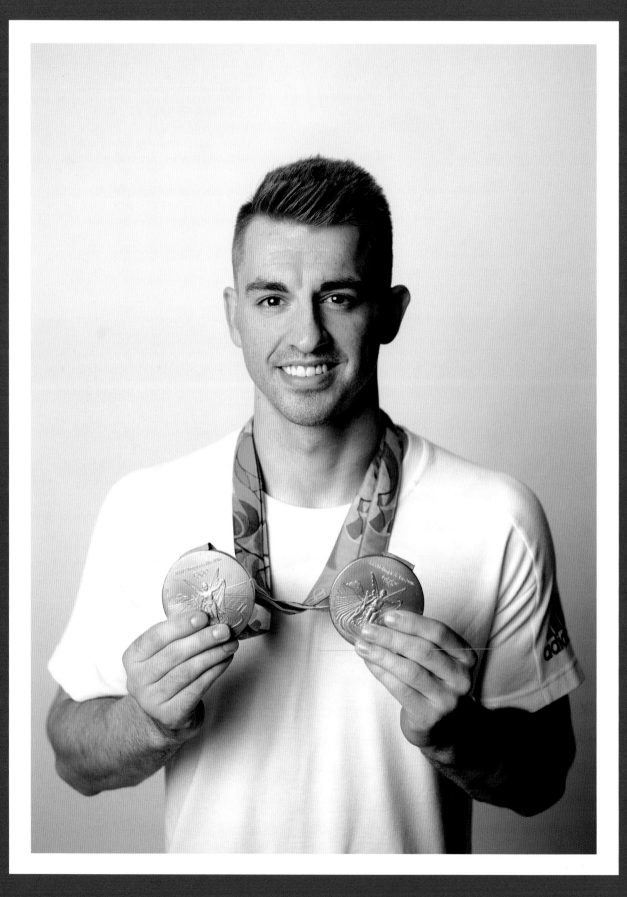

MAX'S LIFE: *MEDAL DAY*

The evening before my gold medal-winning day in Rio I went for dinner in the Athlete's Village. I had my normal pre-event meal of chicken, rice and some broccoli. Simple, easy to digest and nutritious. It's fairly crazy in the Athlete's Village as there are so many athletes from so many countries and competing in such a huge array of sports. It's a huge dining room and you've got some athletes who have finished their events with massive pizzas, and others who have events coming up have tiny little plates mainly composed of salad. I just tried to stay in my zone, stay focused and not to get too distracted by what was going on around me.

After dinner, I went back to my room, had a stretch and then popped down to the physio room for a 10-minute ice bath. After a shower, I was in bed for 2200. I tried not to think about the next day but you can't help but go through routines in your head. No matter how many competitions I've done, I still get nervous but eventually I was able to switch off and get some sleep. I didn't have to be up until 0900 so was still able to get a good 10–11 hours.

It was then back to the Athlete's Village for breakfast and I had my normal tried-and-tested bowl of cereal and a serving of scrambled eggs. Routine and familiarity are so important and the morning of an Olympic final isn't when you want to try something new!

After my breakfast I headed back to my room and went through a stretching routine to try to stay supple, focused but relaxed. I put on my compression gear, just trying to do everything I could to improve my performance, even if only by a per cent, as all of those percentage points add up. I then tried to stay as relaxed as possible until lunch. Again, a meal I've had a thousand times before – pasta, chicken and vegetables – but I know it works for me.

I then headed to the arena. Part of my pre-competition routine, which I know some people disagree with, is I like to use ice bags on my legs and arms before I start warming up. It sounds strange to cool down before warming up and it's probably as much psychological as physical for me, but it seems to make my body feel fresher and lighter. Again, this has just become part of my preparation and routine and it works for me. This then carries through into my final stretches and warm-up, which are exactly the same as I do before every training session at my gym in Basildon. I never watch any of the other gymnasts compete or want to know their scores. I just want to stay in my zone and focus on doing the best routine I can. In doing that, the only person I'm competing against is myself and that takes some of the pressure off. I just sit on my chair, keep my head down and get ready to go.

My actual routine that day is a total blur but the moment that really sticks was finishing it and the sense of relief that brought. I'd done it hundreds of times in training but to hit it perfectly on that one occasion is a big ask. When the realisation hit me that I'd won, it was an unbelievable feeling but a bit delayed as I had no idea what the gymnasts before me had scored or what score I needed to win. The rush of emotions was incredible. I'd watched athletes on TV, seen them bursting into tears but just couldn't imagine that happening to me. It did, though, and those emotions hit me like a tonne of bricks. The culmination of four years of work and expectation just crescendo at that point and something has to give. It all happened so quickly and, within minutes, I had the medal around my neck and was listening to the National Anthem. Crazy.

I didn't get a huge amount of sleep that night as the adrenaline just carried me through. I hid my medal under some clothes and locked it away in my suitcase. It was the next day, though, when the adrenaline stopped, that I realised how much my body ached, how tired I was, but I also had a deep sense of satisfaction.

CARDIO-VASCULAR TRAINING

You'll certainly find that, because of the circuit-style structure of my workouts and the full-body nature of the exercises, your heart and lungs – your cardiovascular (CV) system – will be working hard. If you're performing my workouts three times a week as recommended, especially once you progress to the higher levels, doing any additional cardiovascular training is by no means a necessity.

However, many people do enjoy going out for a walk, run or bike ride, and, as part of a balanced exercise regimen, regular focused CV training can really contribute to health, weight management and overall fitness. If you already run, cycle or do some other CV training, it'll complement my workouts well and you might even find that the strength and mobility my workouts build will improve your performance in those activities.

Almost every Wednesday I'll do a 2-mile run with the aim to do it as quickly as possible. As I get closer to competition, the length of the run will drop and I'll be aiming to sprint as much of it as I can. Most of my routines are 60–70 seconds and I'll try to get the length, and intensity, of the run as close to that of my routines as possible. As with all training, it should be specific to your goals and what you want to get out of it.

SCHEDULING IT IN

You've got a number of options for scheduling in CV training with my workouts:

If you're looking to do 20–30 minutes or so, there's no reason why your CV training can't be an extended warm-up for one of my workouts. If you've done this, you can skip the 2-minute Heart Rate Raiser and go straight into the Neck Rolls and the other mobilisation movements. If you've got a suitable park nearby, you could walk or run to the park, do one of my workouts there and then walk or run home to finish off with my 5-minute Post-workout Stretch Routine (page 36) or, if you have time, my full Stretching/Recovery Routine (page 144).

Another option is to do your CV training on alternate days to my workouts. This can work well, especially if you're training for a CV goal, such as a marathon, triathlon or a sportive cycle ride, and need to do longer sessions. If you adopt this approach, be careful not to overdo things and try to ensure that you schedule in at least one complete rest day each week.

Finally, you can work on a split day, where you'd do my workout in the morning and your CV training in the late afternoon/evening. This can work well if you're already at a good level of fitness, but again don't try to cram too much in and do ensure you have those days off.

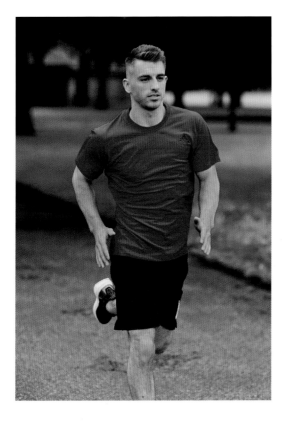
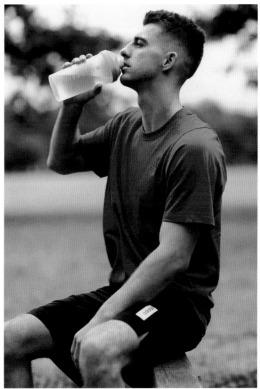

THE FAT BURNING ZONE MYTH

Many pieces of CV kit that you'll find in gyms will either use hand plates or a chest strap, so you can monitor your heart rate while exercising. Invariably these machines will have some form of chart on them or allow you to input your age and give you suggested training zones.

The main problem with this is that training zones based on age-derived formulas are always going to be at best an approximation and are more likely to be wildly inaccurate. If you're interested in training using heart rate, which I'd recommend if you are training for CV-focused goals such as a marathons, sportives or triathlons, there are far more accurate and personalised methods for setting training zones that you can find out more about in specialist books and on websites that cover those activities.

On exercise machines you'll often find a list or chart of zones. There will be a 'fat burning zone' which will be at a relatively low intensity. The reasoning behind this is that at lower exercise intensities our body will use fat as its primary fuel source and, as we up the intensity, it becomes increasingly reliant on carbohydrates. So, you'd think, if you were wanting to lose fat, you should exercise in this 'fat-burning zone'. The problem with this is, because the intensity is so low, unless you exercise for hours on end, your calorie burn will be disappointingly low too. Despite the fact that working harder will almost exclusively burn carbohydrates, even in 20–30 minutes you can burn significantly more calories. Fat loss pretty much comes down to calories in and calories out and, more or less, the form in which you take in and burn those calories is largely irrelevant. So, no matter how appealing it may seem, exercising in the 'fat-burning zone' at an intensity that barely raises a sweat isn't the way to go for fat loss. Up the intensity, do some intervals and work hard!

STRETCHING/ RECOVERY ROUTINE

| TIME: 5–20 MINUTES |
| EQUIPMENT: NONE |

This Stretching/Recovery Routine is my go-to on rest days, after training sessions or if I just feel I need to loosen myself up a bit, such as after a long drive. The 5-minute Post-workout Stretch Routine (page 36) is great if you're pushed for time after a workout but, for a deeper and more focused stretching and mobility session, this routine is really worthwhile. It won't just help you to recover from your previous workouts but, by developing your flexibility, will help you to perform better in subsequent ones. I'd definitely make it a priority on your rest days and, if you're sat in front of the TV in the evening, why not do a bit of stretching?

STRUCTURE

This routine has a simple structure where you just work through the stretches in the order given. You'll find that most of the stretches flow into each other and, once you've done them a few times, the order will feel very intuitive.

However, as we're all different, don't feel that the guidelines are set in stone and, if you want to devote more time to certain stretches than others, go with what feels right for you.

Hold each stretch for 15–60 seconds or, if it feels especially tight, even longer.
Breathe deeply into the stretch and, as the tightness eases, allow the stretch to develop and deepen.
Avoid bouncing or trying to force the stretch.
If you struggle with some of the stretches, for example you might not be able to reach your toes with straight legs, invest in a yoga strap or use a towel to modify the stretch. You can also work with bent knees; do what feels right and works for you.

1. SEATED RELAXATION

Just taking a few moments to relax, focus on your breathing and, if you've been doing a workout, to allow your heart rate to come down.

Sit on the floor with your legs straight out in front and hands on your lap.

Close your eyes, sit up tall, take a few deep breaths and tune in to any particular areas of tightness or soreness that you might have.

When you feel calm, centred and ready, move on to the first stretch.

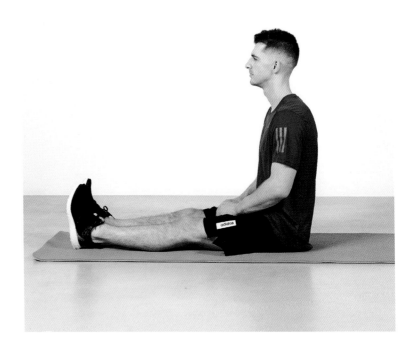

2. FOOT GRAB AND SWEEP

Focusing on your hamstrings and outside of your thighs.

From the seated position, reach forwards with one hand and, keeping your leg as straight as possible, take hold of your toes with the hand on that side.

Slowly elevate that leg, using your other hand to support the back of your thigh.

Move your leg towards the centre of your body, pausing at any sore/tight spots.

Repeat with the other leg.

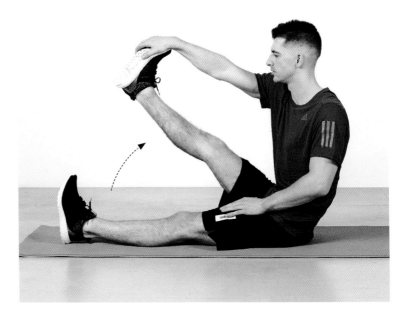

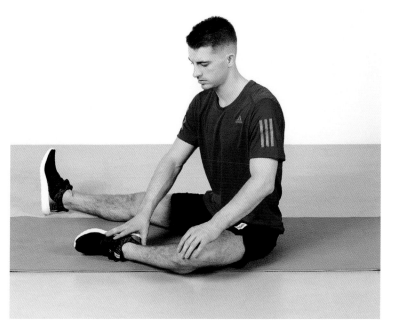

3. BENT LEG FORWARD LEAN

Continuing to stretch your outer thigh but also moving into your buttocks.

Keeping one leg straight, bend the other and allow it to lie flat on the floor with your heel near to your groin.

Supporting your weight with your arms, slowly lower your chest towards the knee of your bent leg.

Repeat on the other side.

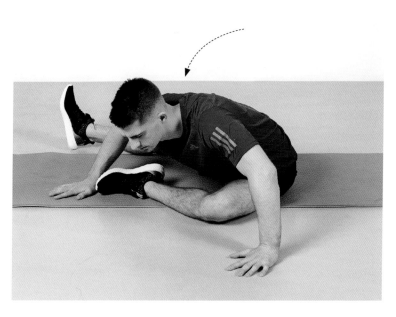

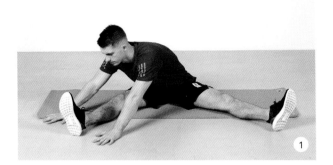

4. STRAIGHT LEG FORWARD LEAN

Hitting the hamstrings and inner thighs.

Sit with both legs straight and out to the sides. Try to find a position where you feel a light stretch in your groin/inner thighs.

Twist and drop your chest forwards towards your knee on one side.

Repeat on the other side.

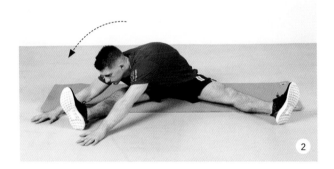

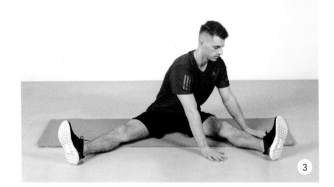

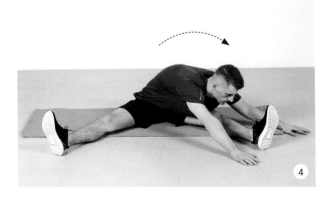

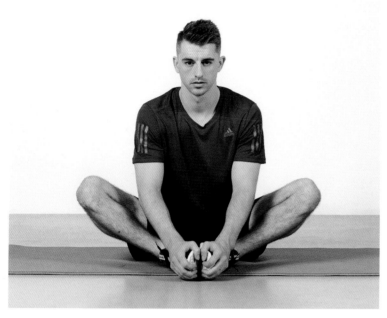

5. BUTTERFLY STRETCH

Moving up into your groin.

Sit with the soles of your feet together and heels close to your groin.

From this position, drop your knees towards the floor.

As tightness eases, gently push down on your knees with your hands to develop the stretch further.

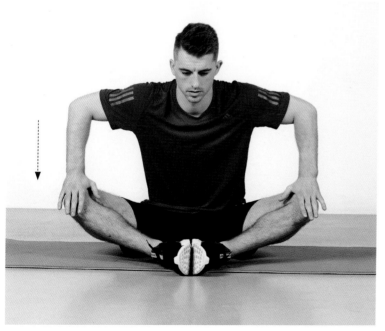

6. BUTTERFLY STRETCH WITH FORWARD LEAN

Taking the previous stretch
a bit further.

Remaining in Butterfly, move
your feet slightly further away
from your groin.

Lean forwards, aiming to rest
your forearms on your shins
and fingers touching toes.

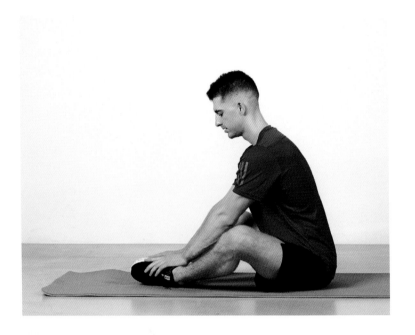

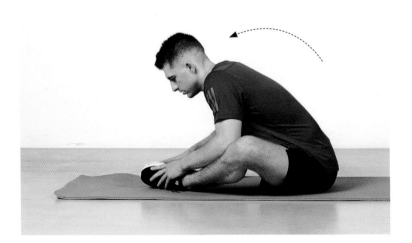

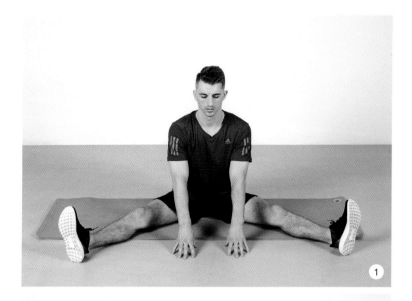

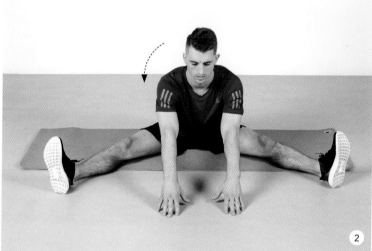

7. JAPANA

With your hamstrings, inner thighs and groin loosened, move on to this challenging stretch.

Straighten your legs out from Butterfly.

Keeping your head up, lean forwards and lower your chest towards the floor.

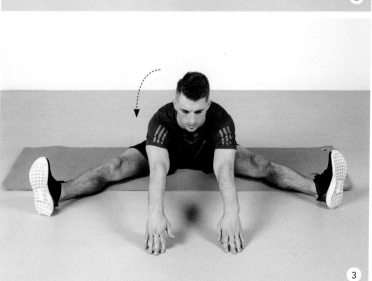

8. QUAD STRETCH

Switching to the front of your thighs and hips. This is a two-phase stretch with the second phase being fairly advanced.

Lying on one side and resting on your elbow, bend your upper leg and, taking your foot in your hand, pull it towards your backside.

If that feels like a good stretch, stay in that position.

If you feel you want to go deeper, roll so that your shin is on the floor and leg tucked to the side. Support your bodyweight on your elbows.

Repeat on the other side.

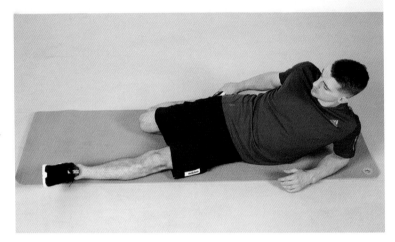

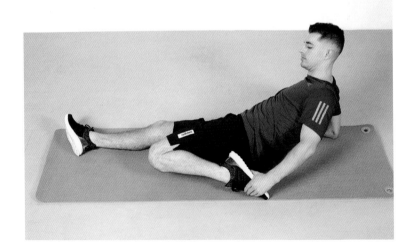

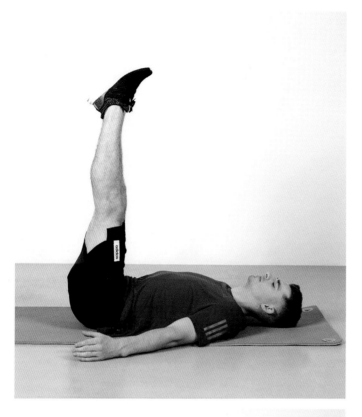

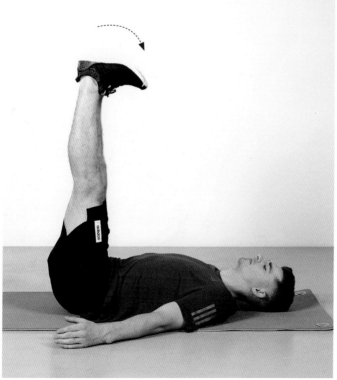

9. LYING ON BACK TOE FLEX

A bit of a breather with this one but it still provides a gentle hamstring, calf and foot stretch.

Lie on your back with your hands behind your head and legs elevated to 90 degrees.

With straight legs, flex and relax your toes and, as you do so, focus again on your breath and on relaxing.

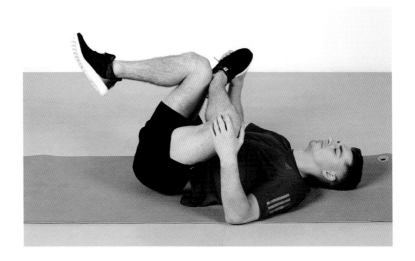

10. GLUTE STRETCH

Another fairly gentle stretch, this time for your glutes.

Staying on your back, bend one leg to 90 degrees and bring the ankle of the other leg to cross it.

You should feel a gentle stretch in your backside.

Repeat on the other side.

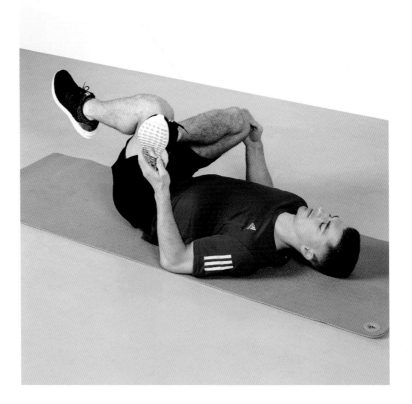

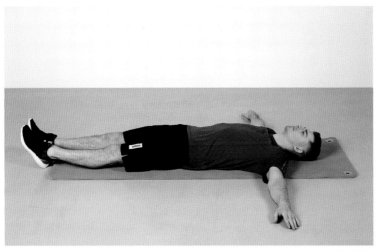

11. ROTATIONAL LOWER BACK STRETCH

A really pleasant-feeling rotational stretch for your lower back.

Still on your back, put your arms out to the side and straighten both legs out.

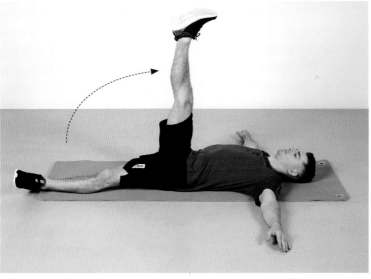

Raise one leg to 90 degrees and then, trying to keep your shoulders square on the floor, cross it over your body and allow it to drop with control towards the floor.

Repeat on the other side.

If you struggle with a straight leg, this stretch is equally good for your lower back with a bent leg.

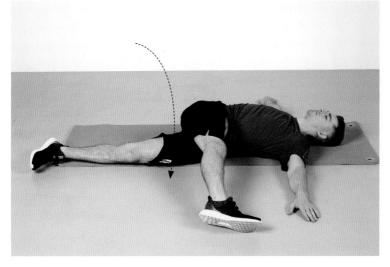

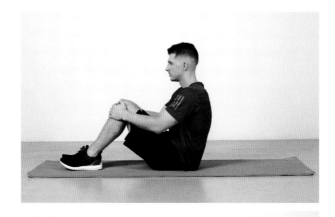

12. ROLLS

A DIY massage for
your spine.

Bring your knees to your
chest, clasp them and lift
your shoulders off the floor.

Rock backwards and
forwards in this position.

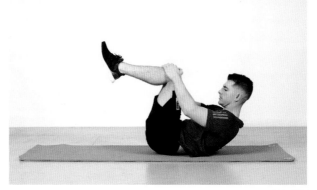

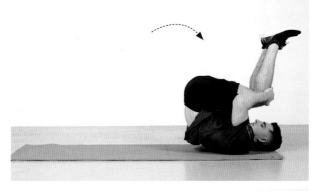

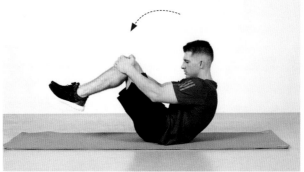

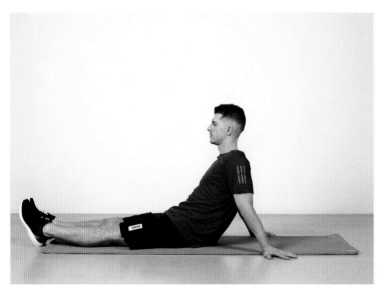

13. LYING SHOULDER STRETCH

Changing the emphasis to your upper body now.

Straighten your legs back out and, leaning back, put your arms behind you with your palms facing down.

Feel a stretch across your shoulders and upper chest and develop it by creeping your hands back.

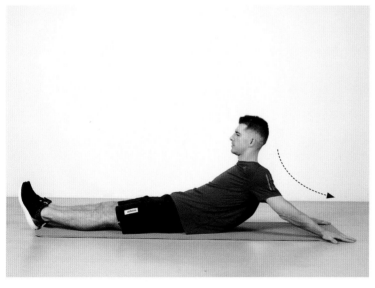

14. WRIST/FOREARM STRETCH

An often neglected but really important stretch, especially if you've been doing any bar or rings work.

This is a 2-position stretch so make sure you do both.

On all fours with your hands facing forwards, rock forwards so that your shoulders go to a position in front of your hands.

Hold this position until you feel you've stretched those muscles enough.

Spin your hands around so that they're facing backwards and sit back onto your haunches.

Hold that position.

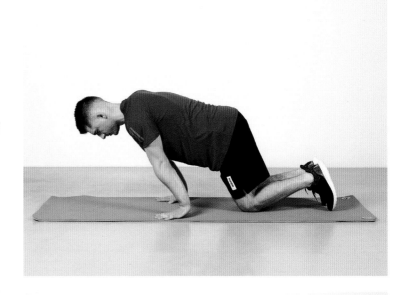

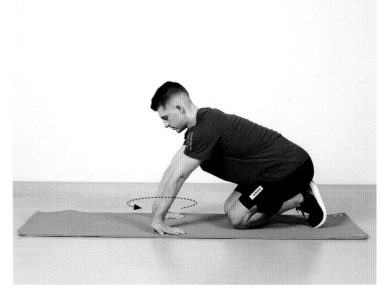

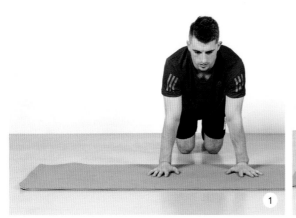

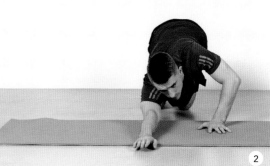

15. SINGLE-ARM SLEEPER STRETCH

Stretching out your lats, shoulders, chest and pecs, which are worked during any pulling movement.

On all fours, reach forwards with one hand and by bending the other arm, twist and drop towards that side.

As the stretch develops, move your arm round to the side to shift the emphasis.

Repeat on the other side.

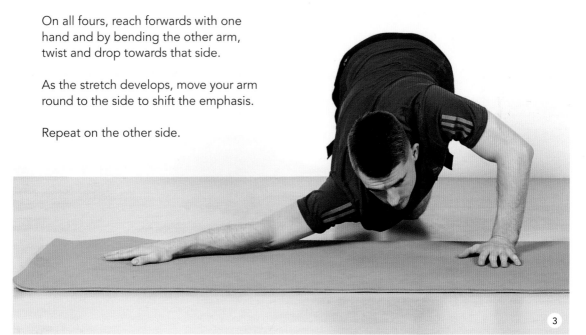

16. SEAL STRETCH

Brilliant for your lower back but will also help your abs recover from sit-up type movements and further stretch your hips and thighs.

Lie face down as if you're going to perform a press-up.

Press-up by straightening your arms but don't allow your groin and legs to come off the ground.

Actively push your groin and legs down as your upper body comes up to create an arch in your lower back.

If this feels too intense, just come up onto your elbows.

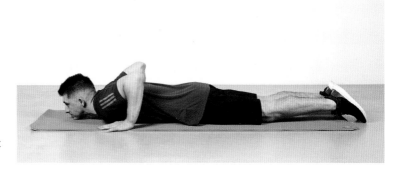

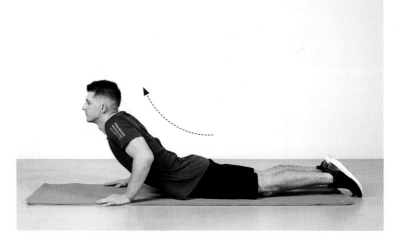

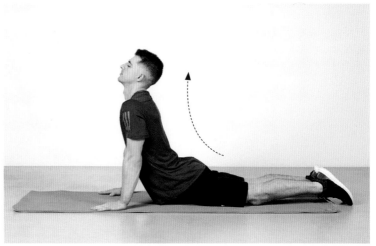

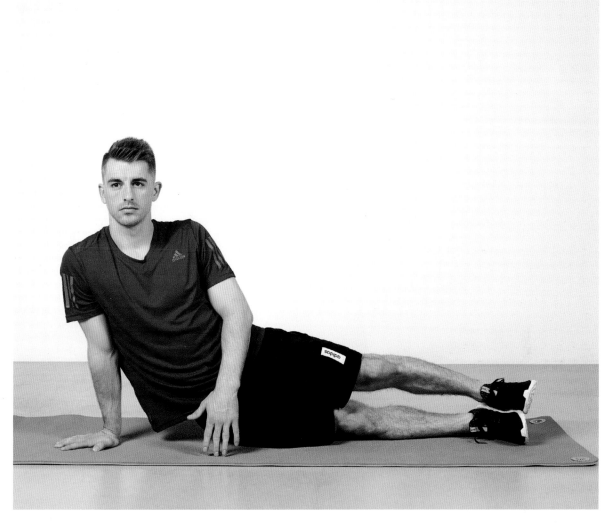

17. SIDE SEAL STRETCH

Stretching the whole of the side of your body from your torso, through your obliques and into your hip and outer thigh.

Lie on one side and, keeping your hips down, elevate your torso off the ground.

Support your weight with your lower arm and use your other arm to aid balance.

Repeat on the other side.

18. CALF STRETCH

A great stretch for runners or if you've been wearing high heels!

Adopt a press-up position with your backside elevated; this is known as Downward Dog in yoga.

Bend one leg and fully straighten the other (think of a sprinter going down on their blocks).

On the straight leg, create a stretch in your calf by pushing your heel down towards the ground.

Repeat on the other side.

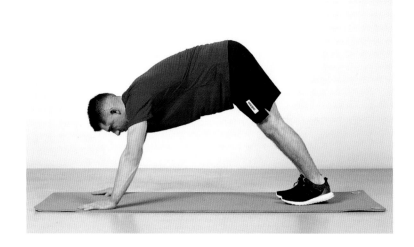

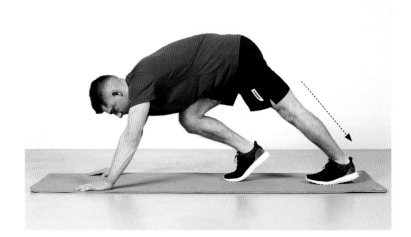

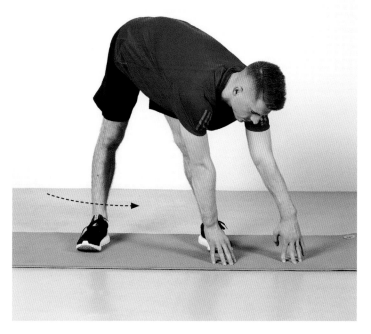

19. STRADDLE TOUCH TOES

Moving up to standing for your hamstrings and lower back.

Stand with your feet wider than hip width apart.

Fold down, dropping your elbows towards the floor.

Bring your hands to the floor and slowly work from side to side, deepening and relaxing the stretch as you encounter tighter areas.

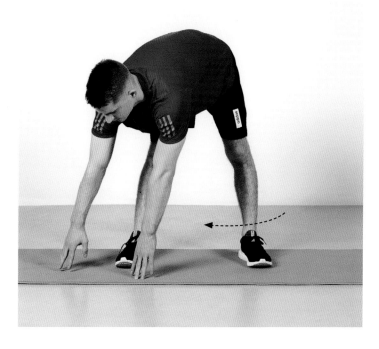

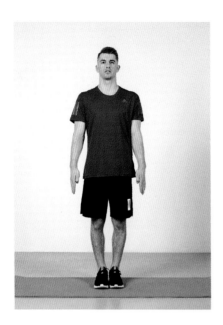

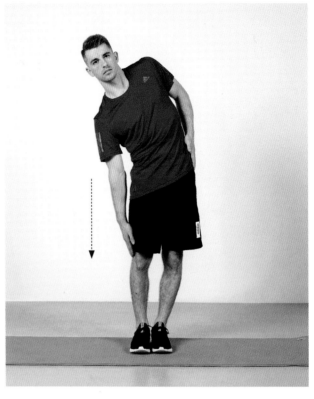

20. SIDE LEANS

Back to your obliques.

Stand with your feet together.

Keeping your torso straight, not leaning forwards or backwards, lean to one side, dropping your hand towards the floor.

Hold your other hand on your hip.

Repeat on the other side.

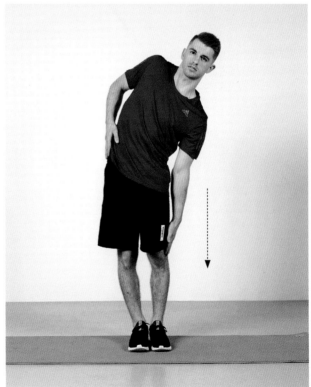

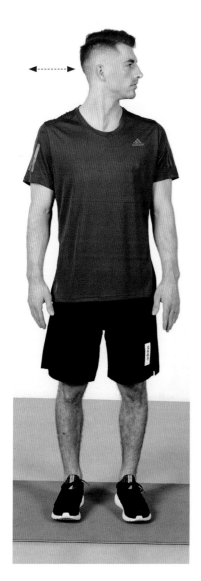
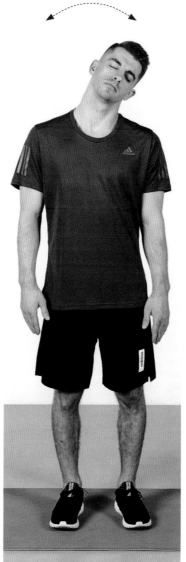
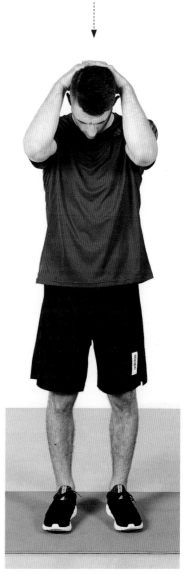

21. NECK STRETCHES

Finishing off with your neck and some deep and focused breathing.

In a standing position, look to the right, hold, back to centre, pause, look to the left and hold.

Drop your left ear to your left shoulder, hold and then repeat on the right.

Drop your chin to your chest, interlace your hands behind your head, gently pull and hold.

Return to centre, shut your eyes and take 5–10 deep and controlled breaths to end the session.

MAX'S LIFE: RECOVERY DAYS

Even now I'm a dad, my rest days are pretty similar to how they've always been; there's just three of us. We'll just chill out, maybe go to the cinema, go and see family and just relax. Around competition times, I'll do some stretching, as that helps me to recover and, in doing that, allows me to train more effectively on Monday and the rest of the week. I've never struggled with switching off and having that rest day as I know it's an essential part of my training.

Always bear this in mind with regards to your own training. Hopefully you'll be really inspired by this book and my workouts but ensure that you build up slowly and don't binge and bust with your training. It's far better to do three quality workouts a week consistently and give yourself those rest days to recharge than trying to train every day and then falling off the wagon exhausted and demotivated after a few weeks.

Any longer periods of time off will be after a major championships. For me, taking that time out and having a holiday is a vital part of my recovery. It allows me to mentally and physically recharge and so is a vital part of my training. Getting away for a week or two gives me the chance for a full switch off. I can then come back rested and ready to build back up again to my full training routine. You can't be on it 100 per cent the whole time or you just stop making progress or burn out.

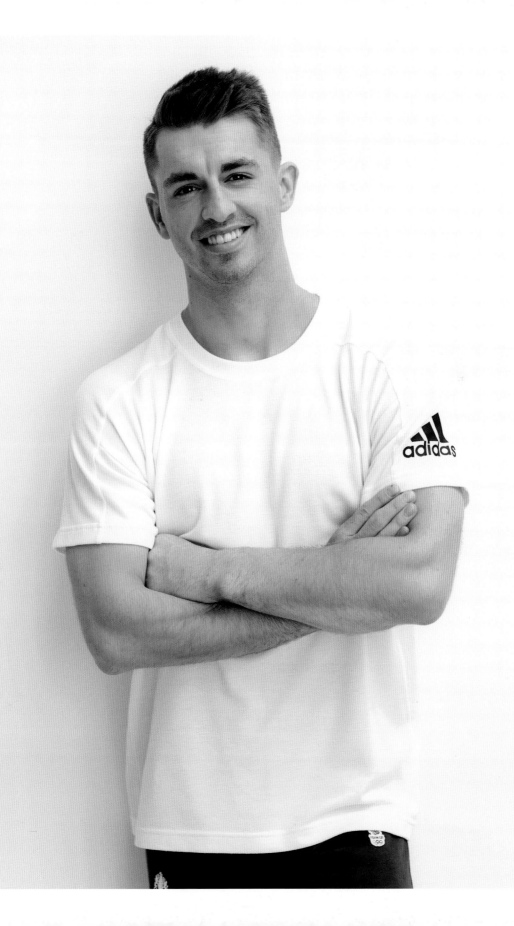

HOW TO BOOST YOUR RECOVERY

I've already stressed the importance of recovery and how it's when you allow your body to recover from training that it gets stronger. Without adequate recovery, you'll not only limit your fitness gains but are more likely to suffer from burnout, possibly injure yourself and be far more likely to slip off the training ladder. It's all too easy, when your start a new training regimen, to get overexcited and overenthusiastic, and this is great, but it has to be tempered in order to develop a sustainable and effective workout habit.

So, my first top recovery tip is to make sure you schedule some in. If you've trained hard one day, don't beat yourself up about chilling out and spending some time lying on your sofa, rather than training on it, the next. Don't forget, you can do some dedicated stretching or some other restorative activity such as Pilates or yoga but try to have at least one complete day off each week.

Make sure you spend some time after each workout cooling down and stretching, as this will start your recovery process and begin to prepare you for your next session.

If you're not going to be having a meal within an hour or so of finishing your workout, have a light snack. This should contain some carbohydrates and some protein. The carbohydrates will re-fuel you and the protein will help your muscles to repair and grow. A glass of milk, it can be soya milk, and a banana is a great option, or one of my Protein Energy Balls (page 251) or some Nut Butter-stuffed Dates (page 248).

Keep well hydrated during the day, during your workout and after it. You don't need to be drinking sports drinks during my workouts but you should have a bottle of water on hand and keep sipping throughout.

I'm also a big fan of compression clothing and the evidence for their recovery benefits is now pretty strong. It's certainly no hardship, if you're chilling out on the sofa after a hard workout or day at work, to slip on a pair of compression tights. They're also great for travelling and make a real difference to how your legs feel after a long drive or flight.

Quality sleep is vital for recovery, getting the most out of your training and for overall health and well-being; I'll always try and get 10–11 hours every night! Long-term poor sleep will also result in diminished mental and physical performance and an increase in the body's stress hormone, cortisol. Try to get into a bedtime routine that is conducive to sleep. Avoid caffeine after 3pm, alcohol and excessive screen time before going to bed – no TV, phone or tablets in the bedroom. Don't perform hard workouts within a couple of hours of going to bed and make sure that your bedroom is well aired, at a comfortable temperature and properly dark.

FOAM ROLLER ROUTINE

30 SECONDS EACH EXERCISE
10 SECONDS REST IN BETWEEN EXERCISES

In an ideal world we'd all have the time and the money for regular massage, as it's a great way to enhance recovery and to keep your soft tissues pliable and healthy. However, using a foam roller offers an easy, cheap and effective DIY option. It's a great option for rest days and a combination of this routine followed by my Stretching/Recovery Routine (page 144) will leave your muscles feeling wonderful. The roller work will release them and then you'll be able to stretch them really deeply. However, this roller routine is also ideal for post workout, either before the 5-minute stretch (page 36) or as a standalone alternative.

BUYING A FOAM ROLLER

There are a multitude of foam rollers on the market, ranging from simple expanded polystyrene to designs that supposedly mimic the action of a therapist's fingers – and even ones that vibrate! The most important considerations are size and firmness. A roller needs to be large enough to be able to effectively perform the movements but not too big, especially if you intend to travel with it. Some models are hollow, which makes them especially suited for travelling as you can pack stuff inside them. Generally, the firmer the roller the better. You'll be putting your entire bodyweight onto it and cheaper or softer rollers will just flex, degrade and won't deliver an effective massage.

WHAT IT DOES

Using a foam roller and a trigger-point ball mimics a therapy technique known as myofascial release. The myofascia is a spider's web-like network of white connective tissue that surrounds all of your muscles. All myofascia are connected and it can almost be thought of as a skin-suit surrounding our muscles. In a healthy state it's soft, flexible and free-moving but repetitive movement, load and trauma can cause it to become tight and unyielding.

STRUCTURE AND GUIDELINES

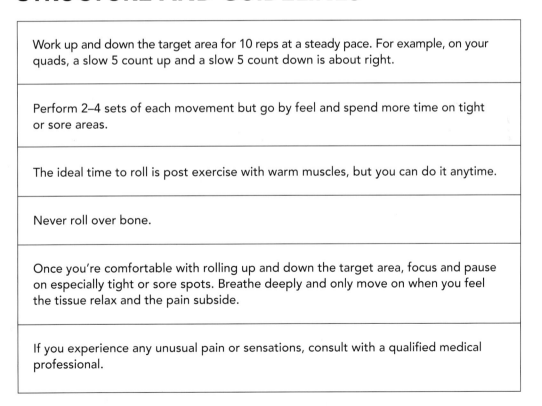

Work up and down the target area for 10 reps at a steady pace. For example, on your quads, a slow 5 count up and a slow 5 count down is about right.
Perform 2–4 sets of each movement but go by feel and spend more time on tight or sore areas.
The ideal time to roll is post exercise with warm muscles, but you can do it anytime.
Never roll over bone.
Once you're comfortable with rolling up and down the target area, focus and pause on especially tight or sore spots. Breathe deeply and only move on when you feel the tissue relax and the pain subside.
If you experience any unusual pain or sensations, consult with a qualified medical professional.

1. SINGLE LEG CALF ROLLS

Start with your calves; pay particular attention to these if you're a runner.

Sit on the floor facing the roller with one leg folded under the other and your top leg with your calf resting on the roller.

Thoroughly roll your entire calf by bending your knee and allowing your leg to rotate both inwards and outwards.

Swap to roll the other calf.

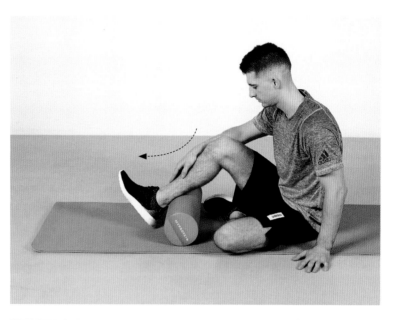

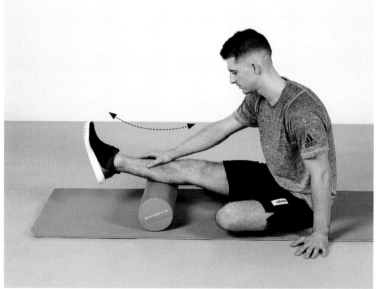

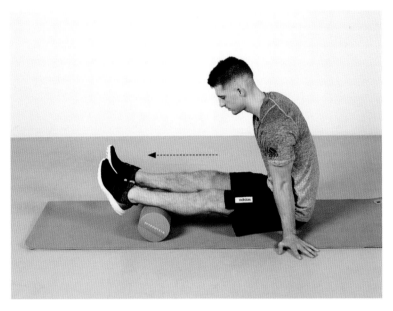

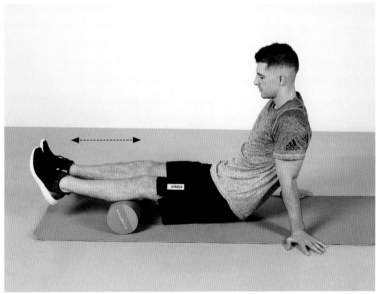

2. DOUBLE CALF ROLLS

With your calves softened and hopefully a bit less sore, you can now move on to rolling with your full bodyweight.

Sit with your legs straight out in front of you, your hands on the floor behind and your calves resting on the foam roller.

Raise your buttocks off the floor so that your weight is supported by your hands and the foam roller.

Roll backwards and forwards along the lengths of your calves.

3. ROLLS BEHIND THE KNEES

Moving up your legs to behind your knees and hitting your upper calves and lower hamstrings.

From the double calf rolls, simply allow the roller to move up behind your knees and focus on that area.

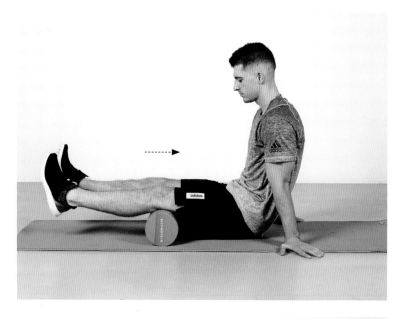

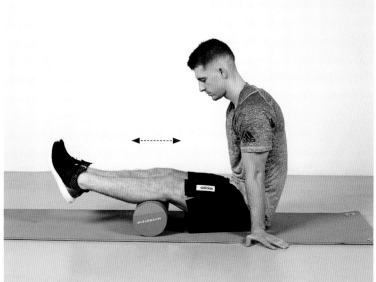

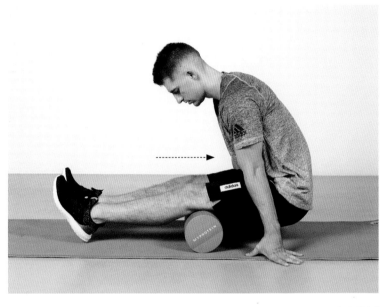

4. HAMSTRING ROLLS

A lot of the exercises in my routines work on improving your hamstring strength and mobility so, as you develop them, they'll need some TLC.

Carry on moving up your legs and now focus on full sweeps from just above your knees to just below your buttocks.

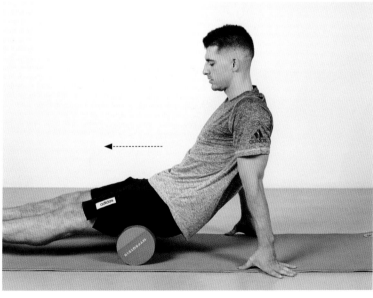

5. GLUTE ROLLS

Your glutes, i.e. your backside, are the biggest and hardest working muscles in your body and so they can get really tight.

Sit on the roller and pivot over so that your weight and focus is on one buttock and then roll it out.

Swap to roll your other buttock.

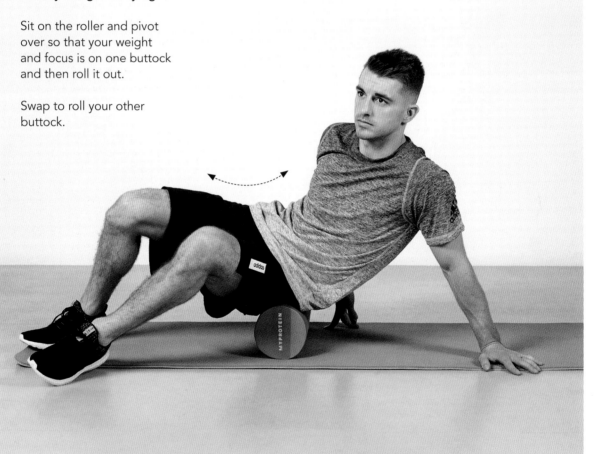

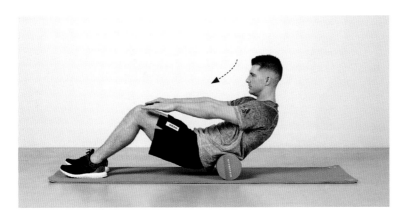

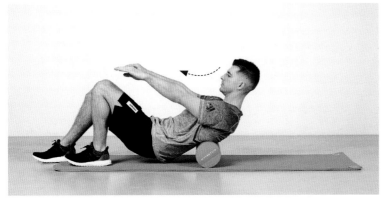

6. BACK ROLLS

Any pulling movement will work your upper back. Also, by loosening off these muscles, you can help rectify any hunched-over posture.

Place the roller underneath your lower back and raise your arms over your head.

Allow the roller to move up further so that you're now working between the top of your lower back and just below your armpits.

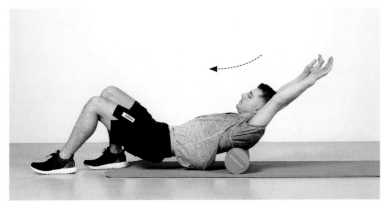

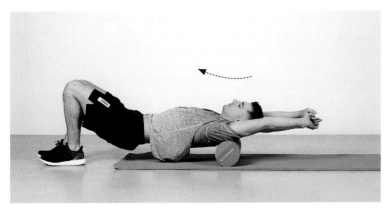

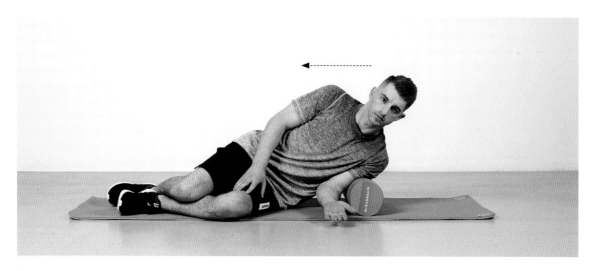

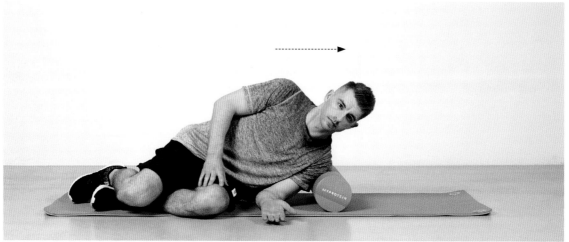

7. SHOULDER ROLLS

On to your upper body now and starting with your deltoids, the muscles on the outside of your shoulders.

Lie on your side with bent legs and your upper leg slightly forwards to aid balance.

Position the roller under the soft tissue of your shoulder and roll from just below the bony prominence to just above your elbow.

Swap to roll the other side.

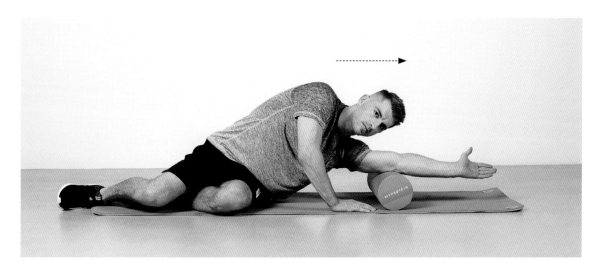

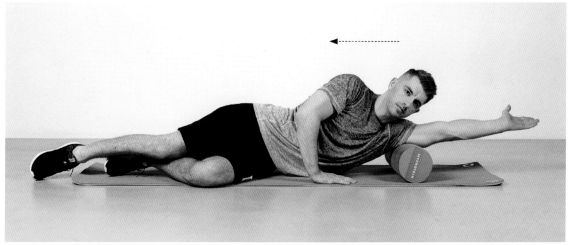

8. TRICEPS ROLLS

If you've done any press-ups or dips then your triceps will need some attention.

Set up with one arm outstretched and on the roller and the other aiding balance and supporting your weight.

Roll from your armpit to just below your elbow.

Swap to roll the other side.

9. PECS AND BICEPS ROLLS

You'll be amazed at how tight and sore your chest can be so take your time with this one and explore those tight spots.

From the triceps rolls position, rotate so that your chest comes onto the roller and extend your arm out to the side.

Roll up and down your chest and vary your arm position to hit your biceps at the same time.

Swap to roll the other side.

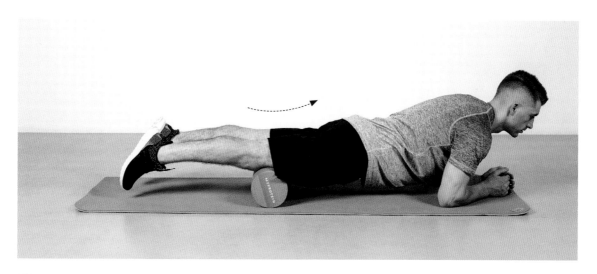

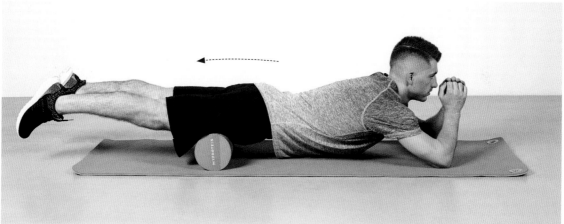

10. QUAD ROLLS

Finishing off with the front of your thighs. This is important if you've done any squatting movements and if you're a runner or a cyclist.

Lie face down in a front plank position with your thighs on the roller and your upper body supported by your elbows.

Roll up and down the full length of your thighs from the top of your hips to just above your knees.

EATING THE WHITLOCK WAY

It's arguable that good nutrition can have a more positive effect on your health than exercise – and poor nutrition a more negative effect. There's a lot of truth in the expression 'you can't exercise away a poor diet'. I'm 100 per cent confident in the effectiveness of my workouts, but if you're not eating well, you won't get all the benefits from them that you should.

My recipes all reflect my no-nonsense, 'no-diet' approach to nutrition; although they undeniably have a healthy slant, they're in no way faddy or low on flavour. Importantly, they're all simple to make and the ingredients are easily available – because I'm definitely no chef!

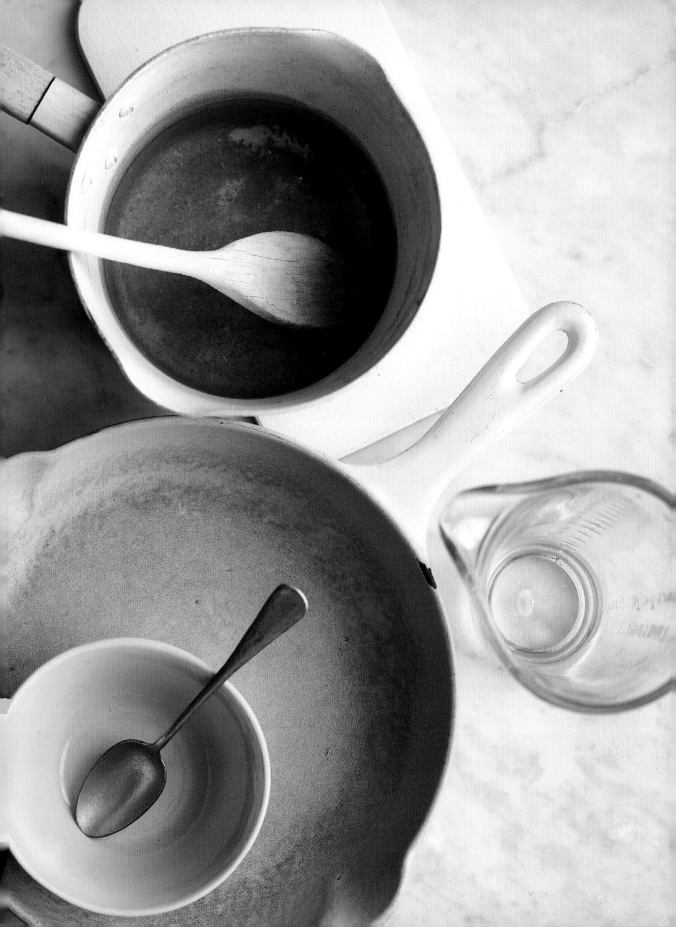

NO-NONSENSE NUTRITION

When I first decided I wanted to write a workout book, it was going to be just that: a book dedicated solely to my gymnastics-focused workouts. However, as I started to put the workouts together, I realised that the main message I wanted to convey was the importance of permanent healthy lifestyle changes, rather than faddy fixes, and this applied equally to nutrition too.

I know what has worked for me over the years and I've also seen some of the weird and wonderful diets that some of my peers have tried. I'm definitely not a salad-and-chicken-breast-only zealot either and believe that a healthy diet can be delicious, fun and not at all restrictive. I've got a real weakness for junk food and you'll see, with a number of my recipes, how I've created healthier twists on popular fast foods to satisfy these cravings.

MY APPROACH TO HEALTHY EATING

THE RULE OF THIRDS

Divide your plate or bowl into:

⅓ protein, such as a chicken breast or similar
⅓ carbohydrates, ideally unrefined, such as wholegrain rice
⅓ salad or vegetables

Obviously, you don't have to fill every third or be 100 per cent precise, it's just about getting the relative proportions about right. Using the chicken breast example again, your carbs and vegetables should occupy a similar amount of room on your plate. There's no need for weighing; it's easy to go on visuals alone.

You'll soon notice that many of your favourite foods and regular meals don't comply with the rule of thirds. Think about some bolognese sauce on a pile of pasta, or a scattering of toppings on a deep-pan pizza. We often tend to overdo the carbohydrates to the detriment of protein and greens. As I've said earlier, carbs aren't evil and definitely don't need to be avoided completely because they are essential for providing fuel. But they do need to be eaten in the correct proportions to protein and fat, and you should cut down on those refined carbs.

If you are looking to lose some weight, especially on days when you're not exercising, you can modify the rule of thirds to:

½ salad or vegetables
¼ protein
¼ carbohydrates

Basically, you're just increasing the amount of salad and vegetables, reducing your total protein and carbohydrate intake but still maintaining the 1:1 protein to carb ratio.

The great thing about the rule of thirds, or its weight-loss variant, is that it's so simple and, once you get used to serving up your meals in the correct proportions, it becomes second nature.

You'll notice that some of my recipes, such as my Healthy Pizza (page 234), don't necessarily follow the rule of thirds. You could balance things up a bit by making sure that the area occupied by salad on your plate is similar to the size of the pizza slices, but this is where my second key guideline comes in.

80:20

The 80:20 rule simply states that approximately 80 per cent of the time you should consciously try to be 'good' regarding your diet and then, 20 per cent of the time, you can give yourself a bit of slack – and cook my healthy pizza!

It's really just putting a number to that old adage 'everything in moderation'. It's so easy to get overwhelmed and confused by all the information – and misinformation – surrounding nutrition but, in reality, as long as you're sticking to whole, unprocessed and unrefined foods the majority of the time, you won't go far wrong.

The 80:20 principle works really well because it means you don't create 'forbidden fruits' and therefore you're far more likely to make positive, sustainable changes to your diet. If you think of twenty-one main meals each week, that gives you four meals when you can break the rule of thirds or treat yourself to something a bit naughty.

Alternatively, you can give yourself a day and a half, maybe Friday afternoon and Saturday, when you're not having to think about your nutrition. Like the rule of thirds, it doesn't have to be 100 per cent precise, it's just a rough guideline to be mindful of and to try to stick to.

It's important that you don't go mad 20 per cent of the time, but I tend to find, by adopting sensible and sustainable healthier eating habits, that you won't feel as though you're on a 'diet' or that you're denying yourself anything – and so it's less likely you will binge out.

MY OTHER HEALTHY-EATING GUIDELINES

Along with trying to stick to the rule of thirds and the 80:20 principle, there are a number of other simple steps and guidelines that'll facilitate sustainable change to healthier eating. You don't need to do all of them all of the time but they're well worth being aware of.

KEEP A FOOD DIARY

I'm not a fan of calorie counting or tracking but if you're trying to improve your diet, keeping a food diary for a few weeks can help. It'll allow you to see where you might be slipping up, as often we can be blind to the dietary hiccups we might be making – that extra biscuit mid-morning or that second glass of wine, for example. Writing down what you eat will make you think about your choices. You can also use a food diary more positively – for example, to ensure that you're eating your minimum of five portions of fruit and vegetables each day.

CHEW

Your grandmother was 100 per cent right when she nagged you to chew each mouthful. Chewing is an important first part of the digestive process; it breaks down the food mechanically but also chemically, via enzymes that are secreted in your mouth. If you rush this first step, your food will leave you feeling less satisfied, you'll get less nutritional value from it and you can get indigestion.

The act of chewing sends messages to your brain to tell the rest of your body that you're eating and you can stop feeling hungry. If you don't chew, you can eat faster than these messages get through, which can lead to overeating.

LOW-HANGING FRUIT

This not only refers to the benefits of eating fruit, but also the easy and obvious dietary changes that can make a big difference.

Cutting out sugary snacks and alcohol, 80 per cent of the time, can have a massive impact. Sugary snacks are incredibly calorie dense but don't tend to be at all filling and are far too easy to mindlessly consume. Along with sugary snacks, sugar-packed soft drinks are an easily avoidable source of empty calories. Just three cans of a typical cola will cancel out your 500-calorie deficit. Similarly, unless you're doing exercise bouts of longer than 90 minutes, you don't need to be drinking energy drinks. Also, although smoothies and juices can be a great way to get some of your five a day, they can also be surprisingly high in sugar and calories. Definitely include them in your diet but don't overdo them.

Alcohol is a double-edged sword. As well as being calorie dense, once you've had a couple of drinks, you're far more likely to make unwise food choices.

SNACK

This might seem counterintuitive but regular snacking is essential for maintaining stable energy levels and preventing overeating at main meals or craving sugar between them. In general, you should be aiming for snacks mid-morning, mid-afternoon and, depending on your activity level, pre- and post-workout and before bed. You can find more advice on timing your snacks when you get to my healthy snacks and treats recipes (see pages 246–63).

AVOID MINDLESS EATING

If you're eating, focus on doing that. Don't watch TV, don't use social media, just sit down and enjoy your food. It might sound old-fashioned but, as with chewing, if you're mindful about your eating, you'll be more aware of what you're consuming and therefore you'll be less likely to overeat. This also applies to snacking, especially in front of the TV or in the cinema. Some popcorn or crisps are fine (remember 80:20), but don't have a huge grab-bag next to you on the sofa that you can just keep dipping into for an entire evening. Put a sensible-sized portion in a bowl and limit yourself to that.

STAY HYDRATED

Our bodies often confuse the sensations of hunger and thirst, so if you've eaten well at your main meals and had your regular snacks but are still feeling hungry, it could well be that you're dehydrated. Before reaching for an extra snack, have a glass of water, give it 10 minutes and see how you feel.

SLEEP AND STRESS

I've already talked about the importance of sleep for recovery (see page 169) and how to improve the quality of your sleep. As I've mentioned, if your sleep is compromised, this will cause an increase in your body's stress hormone, cortisol. A typical 'survival response' to chronic elevated cortisol, along with holding on to fat, is to stimulate appetite because your body thinks it needs more calories to cope. Also, this is strongly tied to a psychological component of seeking comfort foods when we're tired and stressed. Really try to do everything you can to maximise the quality of your sleep and to limit factors and behaviours that compromise it.

EAT TO FUEL WHAT YOU'RE DOING

Don't fall into a rut of eating exactly the same meals every day. Not only will this make your diet boring and be more likely to lead to mindless eating, it also doesn't take into account the activity you're doing. On days when you're exercising, you'll probably need more carbohydrates to fuel that activity, but on a rest day, you'll want to put more of an emphasis on protein.

PLAN

Probably the most significant step to improving your diet is to plan ahead and be organised. Plan ahead your meals each week and shop accordingly. This will prevent you running out of food, coming home to empty cupboards or reaching for the takeaway menu. When you cook, get into the habit of making extra portions and building up a stock of meals in your freezer or having one for your lunch the next day. Pack your lunch and snacks to take to work and this will help you to avoid snacking on biscuits and cakes or trips to the sandwich shop.

MAX'S LIFE: MY DAILY DIET

I normally get up at about 0900 and, although this is fairly late, a decent amount of sleep is so important to me and my ability to train, recover and ultimately compete. I'll then have breakfast at about 1000 and aim to get a decent balance of carbs and protein. For me, breakfast is all about providing me with enough energy to keep me going through training but I don't want anything too heavy. I might opt for smashed avocado on toast with a poached egg or some cereal as well as some scrambled egg or an omelette. I'll also make sure I have water so I'm starting the day well hydrated.

It'll be between 1100 and 1200 before I get to the gym and start training and, before that, I'll normally have a small snack to keep my energy levels up. Again, I don't want to feel weighed down or heavy during my workout but I also don't want to feel weak or that my stomach is empty. So it'll just be something like a banana, an apple and maybe some nuts. I'll then typically train for 3–4 hours depending on the time of year and what phase of training I'm in. I'll keep sipping on fluids throughout the workout.

It's fairly late for lunch by the time I finish training but, as I only live ten minutes from my gym, I can at least get the recovery process started fairly quickly and that's what lunch is all about for me. It'll tend to be a really balanced plate of food with carbs, protein and plenty of vegetables. I'll also often have a glass of milk for some extra protein. If I'm training or competing away from home and might not be able to eat so quickly after my session, I'll have a protein shake as soon as I finish training to kickstart my recovery and see me through to lunch.

My lunch is normally fairly substantial and, being so late, I don't always need a snack in the afternoon or early evening. However, if I am a bit peckish, I'll go for something light, such as more fruit, nuts, a Protein Energy Ball (page 251) or Nut Butter-stuffed Dates (page 248).

I'll have my dinner at about 2000, which is again quite late. The main reason my meal timings are a bit strange is that it synchs well with how and when I'd eat during a competition. This means that I'm always in this rhythm and routine and don't have to make any changes or transitions; it's all about finding that extra 1 or 2 per cent in performance gains. Dinner, like lunch, will be well balanced in terms of macronutrients and I try to follow the rule of thirds.

During competition time, when I'm training really hard, I'll often have a light snack before bedtime, such as yoghurt. It provides some slow-release protein to help recovery during the night but doesn't make me feel bloated or interfere with the quality of my sleep.

I'm only human and definitely sometimes crave something a bit naughty. I love cakes and a bit of chocolate. I don't see the point in denying these cravings and find, if I allow myself the odd treat, that the cravings don't become overwhelming. I'll try, where possible, to go for healthier options. If I fancy some chocolate, for example, I'll opt for some with a higher cocoa content or some chocolate-covered raisins.

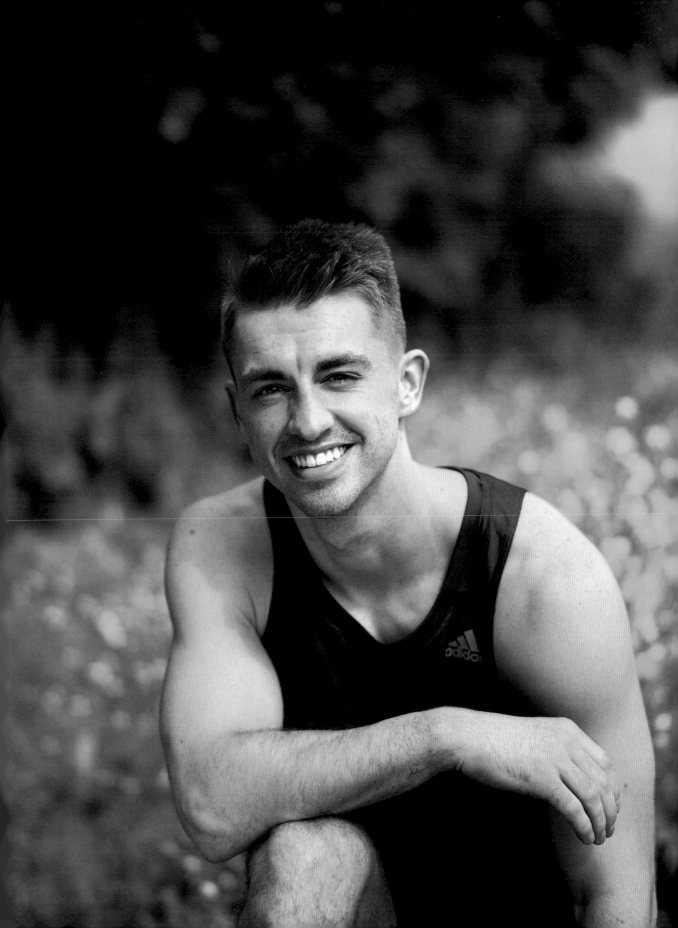

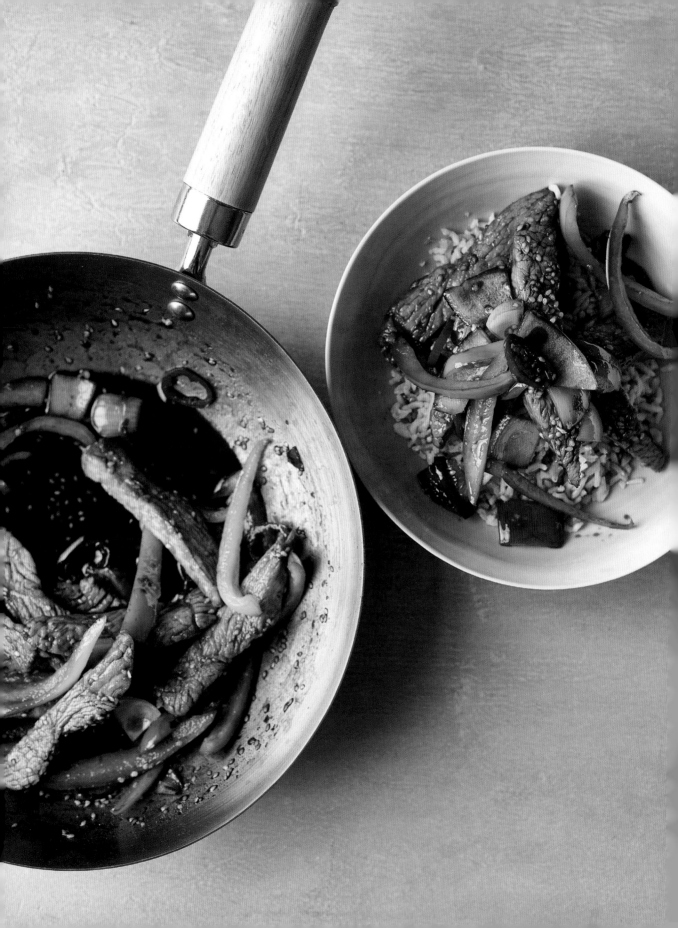

RECIPES INTRODUCTION

The best way to eat more healthily is to prepare your own meals as much as possible. Yes, you can now get some healthy and delicious ready meals and takeaways, but by making the effort to cook for yourself, you're completely in control of what you're eating. If you've cooked a meal yourself, there's no doubt that you'll appreciate it more, eat it more mindfully and find it far more satisfying than something you've just popped in the microwave and eaten in front of the TV. This can help with feeling fuller and more satisfied after your meal and reduce cravings for sugary snacks in the evenings. Cooking for yourself, although perhaps requiring a bit more time and organisation, is also good for your bank balance, especially if you can freeze portions or roll dinners over to the next day. I love cooking for myself, Leah and Willow and then eating together as a family. Dinner time gives us all a chance to properly catch up. It's one of my favourite times of the day.

With these 28 recipes – 7 breakfasts, 7 lunches, 7 dinners and 7 snacks and treats – I've tried to include as many of my personal favourites as possible. I particularly like the recipes that take a junk food or takeaway classic and give it a healthy twist, such as my Thai-style Turkey Burgers, Healthy Pizza and Healthy Fish and Chips (see pages 230, 234 and 238). When I make these for myself, my family and friends, it feels like we're having a bit of a naughty treat, when, in reality, it's a healthy and nutritious meal. Importantly, they're all simple to make and the ingredients are commonly available in all good supermarkets.

I've also provided the carb, protein and fat content of each recipe, as well as the number of calories. Any additional servings (such as rice, bread etc.) aren't included in the nutritional information.

BREAKFASTS

We have all heard the 'breakfast is the most important meal of the day' cliché, but for me it's 100 per cent true. A decent breakfast lays the foundations of my day, whether I'm training, having a rest day or competing. I know that if I have a good breakfast, with carbs, protein and healthy fats all represented, it'll see me through to my mid-morning snack and I'll be far less likely to be tempted by sugary treats to give me a boost.

Many of the breakfasts here are suitable for busy weekday mornings, and the Overnight Oats and the Egg Muffins especially are brilliant if you tend to be a bit rushed and harassed first thing. My Healthier Eggs Benedict and Huevos Rancheros are more suited to chilled weekend brunches or holidays and, although still healthy and nutritionally sound, feel like a real treat.

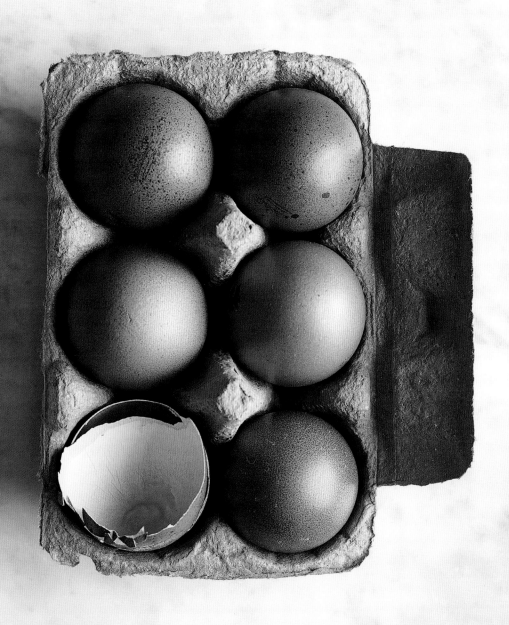

SMASHED AVOCADO ON TOAST WITH POACHED EGGS

(VEGETARIAN)

SERVES 1

2 tbsp white wine vinegar

2 eggs

1 thick slice of bread
  (wholegrain is best)

½ ripe avocado,
  peeled and destoned

splash of Tabasco (optional)

salt and pepper

This is one of my favourite breakfasts because it delivers all the macronutrients and, despite feeling fairly luxurious and a bit of a treat, is really quick and easy to make. It's a brilliant option if you've done a tough pre-breakfast workout. It's also super filling and, with the protein from the egg and healthy fats from the avocado, will easily keep you going until your mid-morning snack.

Add the vinegar to a small, shallow pan of water and bring to the boil. The vinegar is the secret to perfect poached eggs and there's no need to swirl the water around. Turn the heat right down and carefully crack the eggs into the water. Leave them to cook for about 2–3 minutes.

While the eggs are cooking, pop your bread into the toaster. When it's done, mash the avocado onto it using a fork.

Using a slotted spoon, carefully remove the eggs from the pan and place on top of the avocado.

Season to your taste. I sometimes like a splash of Tabasco for a bit of a spicy kick.

PER SERVING

KCALS	354
CARBS	21g
PROTEIN	18g
FAT	22g

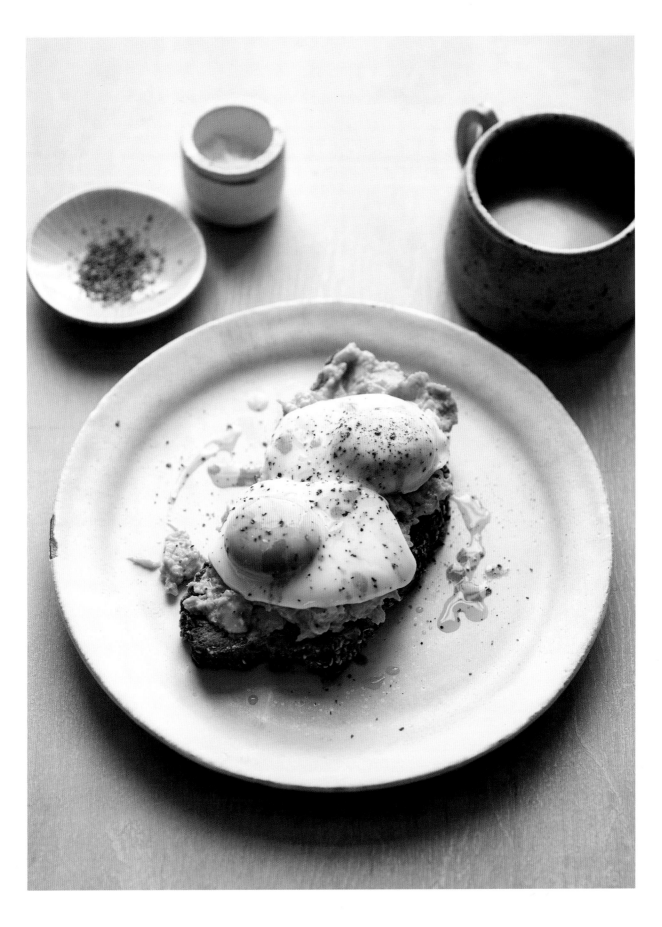

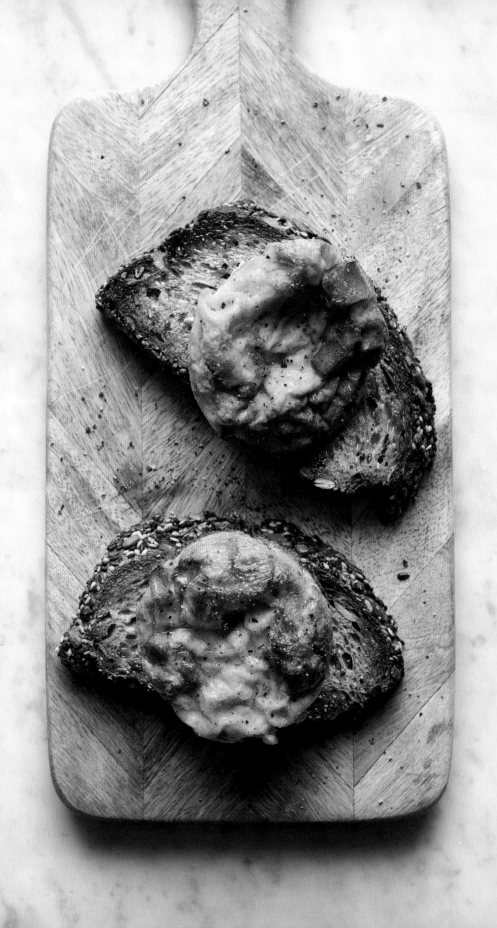

EGG MUFFINS

MAKES 12 MUFFINS

olive oil, for greasing

12 eggs

120ml skimmed milk

6 slices of ham, diced

salt and pepper

wholegrain toast, to serve

Many people skip breakfast or opt for unsatisfying choices, such as cereal or toast, because they feel rushed in the morning and don't think they have time for anything more substantial. The great thing about these muffins is that you can make a batch at the weekend, stick them in the fridge and then just zap them in the microwave for a fast, filling and protein-packed breakfast. You could also add other ingredients to mix things up, such as tomatoes, mushrooms or spinach leaves.

Preheat the oven to 180°C/gas mark 4 and lightly grease a 12-hole muffin tin with olive oil.

In a large bowl, vigorously whisk together the eggs and milk until you've worked plenty of air in. Stir in the ham and season with a little salt and pepper.

Divide the egg mixture evenly between the holes of the muffin tin, then place the tin in the oven and bake for 25–30 minutes, or until the eggs are set.

Once the muffins are baked, allow to cool before removing from the tin.

Store them in an airtight container in the fridge for up to a week. To reheat, simply microwave for 60 seconds.

Serve with some buttered wholegrain toast.

PER SERVING
(toast not included)

KCALS	184
CARBS	1g
PROTEIN	19g
FAT	11g

COCONUT MILK QUINOA PORRIDGE
(VEGAN)

SERVES 1

50g quinoa flakes

150ml coconut milk

2 tsp coconut oil

agave nectar, to taste

Porridge is a brilliant warming breakfast for cold winter mornings. This vegan-friendly version uses the so-called 'superfood' quinoa instead of traditional oats. All of the claims about quinoa might not quite stack up but it is tasty and a great plant-based source of protein. The coconut milk and oil also have a number of health benefits and provide additional slow-release energy. Try adding seeds, nuts or berries too.

In a breakfast bowl if using a microwave or a saucepan if cooking on the hob, stir together the quinoa flakes and coconut milk. You can do this step the night before so it's ready to go in the morning.

In the microwave, cook for about 3 minutes on full power, remove, stir, then cook for another 2 minutes. Repeat until the grains are soft. This should take about 10 minutes in total.

On the hob, bring the quinoa and coconut milk to the boil, reduce the heat to low, cover and cook for approximately 10 minutes, stirring frequently, until the grains are soft.

Before serving, stir in the coconut oil and drizzle with agave nectar, to taste.

PER SERVING

KCALS	308
CARBS	40g
PROTEIN	7g
FAT	14g

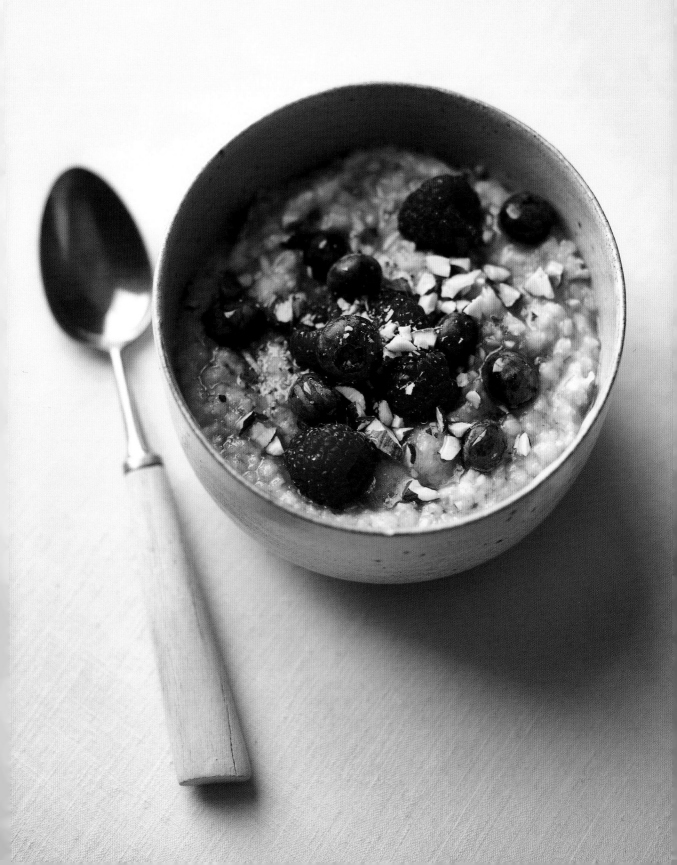

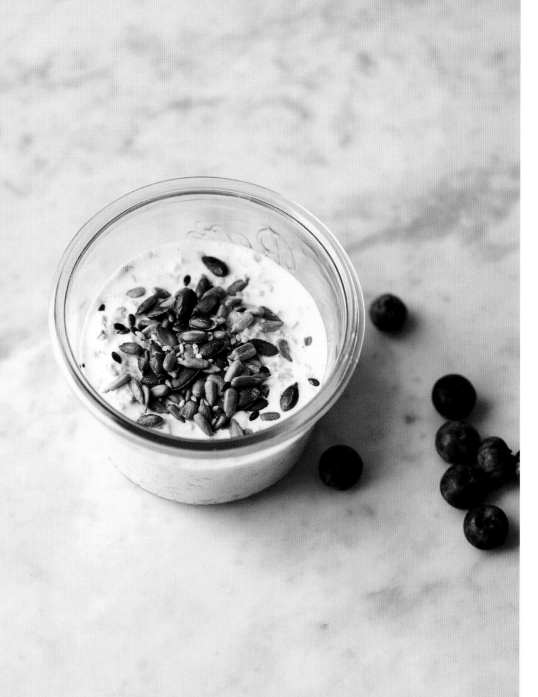

OVERNIGHT OATS

(VEGETARIAN)

SERVES 1

30g rolled oats

80ml milk of your choice

85g Greek yoghurt

protein powder (optional.
I like My Protein)

nuts and seeds (optional)

Sometimes you just know that your morning is going to be a rush, but there's no excuse not to have a decent breakfast. With minimal prep the night before, these Overnight Oats will be ready and waiting in the fridge to deliver both slow- and fast-release carbs as well as a protein hit. Feel free to top with nuts, seeds, honey, fruit or anything else you fancy.

Stir the ingredients together in a bowl or other container. You could stir in a scoop of protein powder or some nuts and seeds if you want at this stage.

Place in the fridge overnight.

In the morning, add any other toppings and enjoy.

PER SERVING

KCALS	258
CARBS	27g
PROTEIN	11g
FAT	11g

with 25g unflavoured whey
My Protein powder and
30g mixed nuts and seeds

KCALS	561
CARBS	32g
PROTEIN	43g
FAT	28g

PROTEIN PANCAKES
(VEGETARIAN)

SERVES 1

2 eggs

1 ripe banana

25g protein powder
(I like My Protein)

1 tsp coconut oil

I love these pancakes because, despite feeling like a bit of a treat, they're actually really healthy, and packed with protein. Plus, you can add all sorts of tasty toppings to them. Try Greek yoghurt, fruit, nuts, agave nectar, maple syrup or whatever else you fancy. They're also really good as a 'take-out' breakfast because they're delicious cold too.

Using a food processor or hand blender, mix the eggs, banana and protein powder together well in a bowl.

In a frying pan, heat up the oil over a medium heat and, using a ladle, add a third to a half of the batter to the pan.

Allow the batter to cook until you see bubbles coming through and then flip it over. This is usually a couple of minutes but keep an eye on them because the fruit sugar in the banana means they can burn quite easily.

Remove from the pan, set aside and cook the next one. You'll probably get around 2–3 pancakes depending on how big you make them.

Then add your choice of toppings and enjoy.

PER SERVING
(without toppings)

KCALS	428
CARBS	30g
PROTEIN	37g
FAT	19g

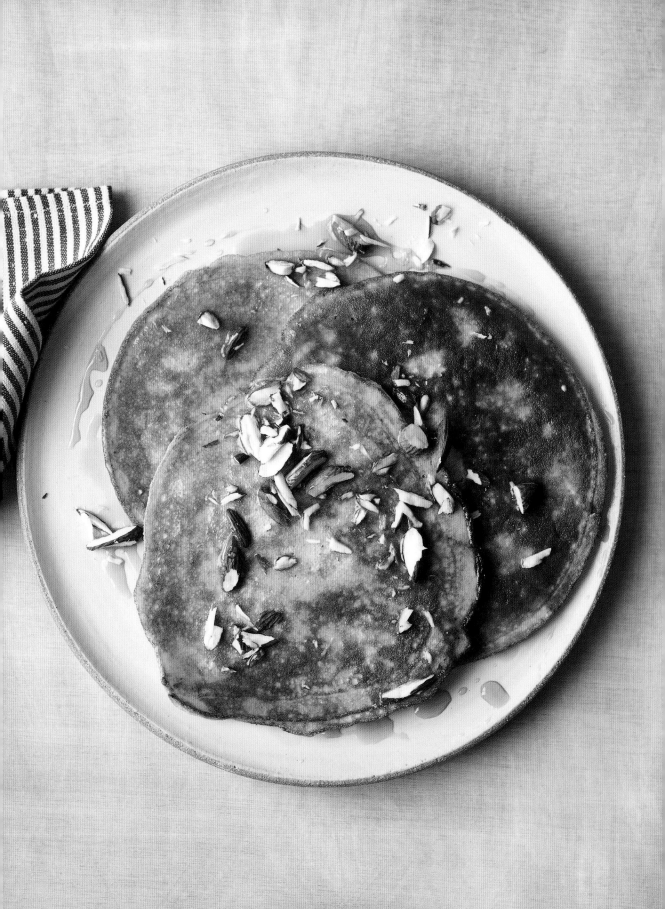

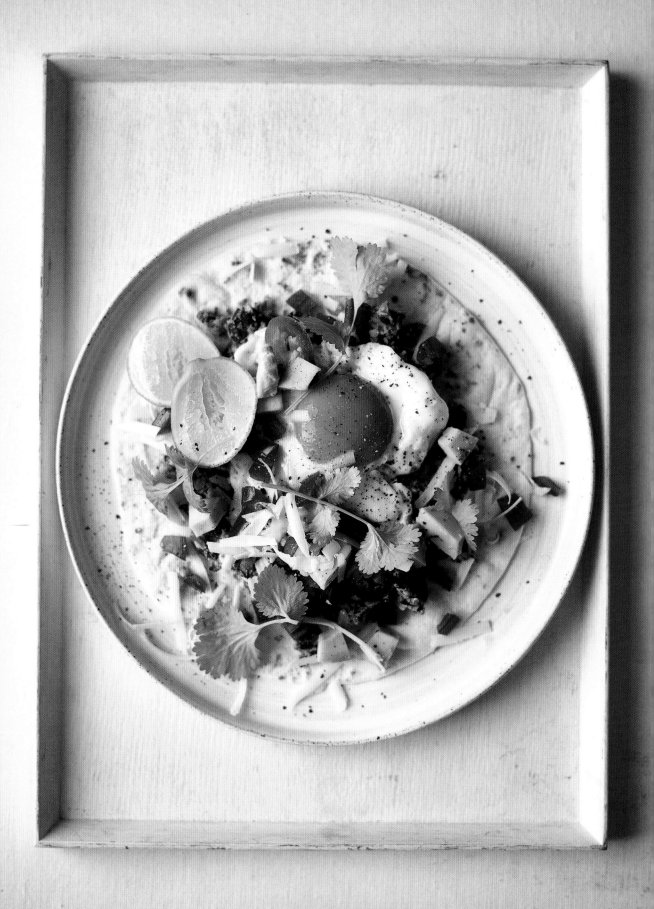

HUEVOS RANCHEROS

(VEGETARIAN)

SERVES 4

4 soft flour tortillas

1 large tomato, diced

½ a 125g jar of pickled sliced
  jalapeño peppers, drained

1 ripe avocado, peeled,
  destoned and diced

juice of ½ lime

2 tbsp olive oil

1 medium onion, diced

2 garlic cloves, crushed

1 x 400g tin of red kidney beans,
  drained and rinsed

1 tsp ground cumin

¼ tsp chilli powder

½ tsp dried oregano

100ml water

4 eggs

30g Cheddar cheese, grated

a handful of fresh coriander,
  finely chopped

salt and pepper

This isn't really a weekday breakfast, unless you have a lot of time in the mornings, but it is perfect for a lazy weekend brunch and is a healthier alternative to a traditional fry-up if you've got friends or family round. This is why this recipe serves four. I love it when I have a rest day and this dish is ideal for fuelling my recovery because it contains good amounts of protein and healthy fats.

Preheat the oven to 170°C/gas mark 3. Stack your tortillas, wrap them in foil and pop them in the oven.

Put the diced tomato, jalapeños and avocado into a large bowl, add the lime juice and some salt and pepper, then give everything a good toss and set aside.

Heat 1 tablespoon of the olive oil in a large pan over a medium heat, add the onions and cook until they start to soften, about 3–4 minutes.

Add the garlic and cook for 1 minute more.

Add the beans, cumin, chilli powder, oregano and water, then season and give everything a good stir.

Cook for 5–7 minutes, stirring occasionally and, once the beans have softened, remove from the heat. Mash well with the back of a fork and set aside.

Heat the second tablespoon of oil in another large frying pan over a medium heat and fry the eggs for a few minutes.

While the eggs are cooking, get the tortillas out of the oven.

Spread the bean mixture onto the tortillas, follow it with the tomato, jalapeños and avocado salsa, top with a fried egg and sprinkle on some Cheddar. Finish with some fresh coriander before serving.

PER SERVING

KCALS	511
CARBS	45g
PROTEIN	20g
FAT	25g

HEALTHIER EGGS BENEDICT

4 SERVINGS

2 tbsp white wine vinegar

4 eggs

4 muffins

butter, for spreading (optional)

4 thick slices of smoked ham

2 tbsp chopped parsley

For the hollandaise

125g full-fat natural yoghurt

1 tsp English mustard

¼ tsp cayenne pepper

salt and pepper

Another lazy Sunday brunch option that you can make for a bunch of mates and enjoy with the weekend papers. I love eggs benedict and hollandaise sauce is one of my real out-of-competition treats. There's no denying that it is high in fat, though, so this healthier option substitutes the butter for yoghurt. For eggs royale, replace the ham with some smoked salmon, or with some wilted spinach leaves for vegetarian-friendly eggs florentine.

To make the healthier hollandaise, simply stir together the yoghurt, mustard, cayenne and some salt and pepper in a small saucepan over a low heat. Warm it through but be careful not to overheat it or it'll split, then take off the heat, put a lid on to keep it warm and set aside.

Follow the egg poaching instructions from the Smashed Avocado on Toast with Poached Eggs recipe (see page 194).

While the eggs are poaching, split and toast the muffins. Butter the toasted muffins if you want and add a slice of ham to one half of each muffin.

Carefully place the poached eggs on top of the ham.

Finally, pour the hollandaise over the top of both muffin halves and sprinkle on some fresh parsley.

PER SERVING

KCALS	327
CARBS	32g
PROTEIN	22g
FAT	11g

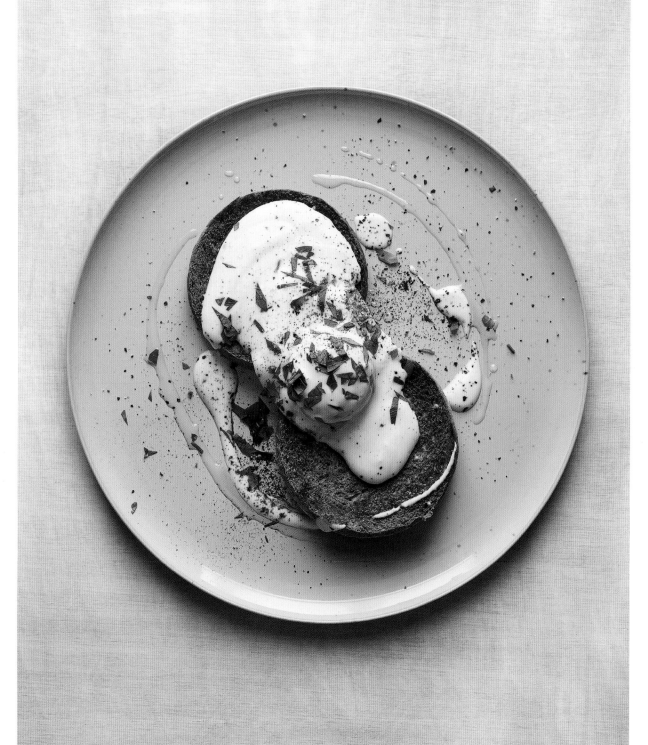

THE
SCALES
DO LIE

If I could urge you to do one thing for your health, fitness and appearance, it would be to ditch your scales. Weight-loss goals are just so demotivating, especially if you're not meeting them, and your weight is not a stable or reliable measurement to track your progress by.

Your weight can vary during the course of a single day by up to 2kg, due to factors such as hydration, how well stocked your body's energy stores are and how much food you have processing in your digestive tract. Yes, you can account for this to an extent by weighing yourself at the same time each day, but there can be a margin of error.

Also, especially if you're exercising, fat loss may not mean weight loss and, if you're gaining muscle, you can even see your weight going up because fat is less dense than muscle. Compare the size of a pound of butter to a pound of lean steak. You can easily be getting leaner and smaller but this won't be reflected by your scales.

It's far better to monitor your body composition by taking some measurements with a tape measure. Hips and waist are good, or simply notice how your clothes feel.

Best of all, though, is just to accept that if you're eating well and exercising, your body will change and, rather than using aesthetic goals, use tangible and achievable exercise and nutritional goals to motivate you. I guarantee you'll be happier, healthier and far more likely to maintain a healthy lifestyle.

LUNCHES

Lunchtime can be really tricky as, more often than not, you'll be at work or, in my case, at the gym. It's all too easy to end up relying on ready-made lunches from the supermarket or sandwich shop chains. As well as being expensive, they're often not the healthiest options. You can also fall into a rut of eating the same lunch every day with no consideration given to your activity that day or your body's needs. If you're bored with your food, you'll tend to eat it mindlessly and that can lead to feeling unsatisfied and overeating later in the day.

All of these lunch recipes can be made fresh and eaten hot but are ideal for making the night before, packing up and having the next day. Buy yourself a few airtight containers and, as long as you have a fridge at work, you're sorted. Each recipe makes two servings so you've either got two days' worth of lunches or you could make it for supper and have the leftover portion the next day for lunch. Also, many of these recipes share ingredients so, say you use half a red pepper for the Chicken and Mango Wraps (page 212), you could use the leftover half for my Vegetable and Bacon Frittata (page 215).

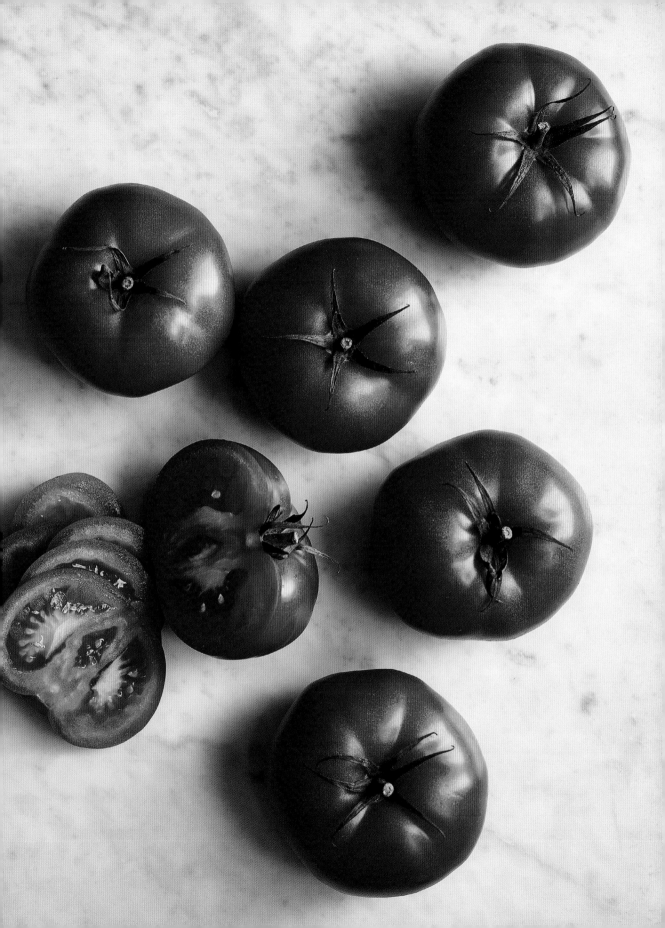

CHICKEN AND MANGO WRAPS

SERVES 2

1 tbsp peanut oil

250g chicken breast,
  cut into strips

½ tsp finely chopped
  fresh ginger

1 tbsp hoisin sauce

100g fresh mango slices,
  or tinned (just drained off)

½ small cucumber, finely sliced

½ red pepper, finely sliced

½ yellow pepper, finely sliced

juice of ½ a lemon

1 tbsp runny honey

½ fresh chilli, deseeded
  and finely sliced

2 tsp sesame seeds

a generous handful of
  mixed salad greens

4 wraps

I love wraps for lunch because you can pack them with delicious ingredients but they're not as heavy as a traditional sandwich. This simple Chinese-style filling is really tasty and, along with the protein from the chicken, has loads of nutrients from the fresh vegetables and, of course, the mango. It's also a great salad on its own or you can combine it with some cooked rice or noodles. Try to get hold of some peanut oil for stir frying as it has a high smoke point and so is suited to high temperatures; it adds a great flavour too.

Heat the oil in a non-stick wok over a high heat. Add the chicken and stir-fry for about 3–5 minutes or until the chicken is no longer pink when cut with a knife.

Add the ginger and the hoisin sauce and cook for 30 seconds, stirring vigorously. Remove from the heat and transfer the chicken to a large salad bowl. Allow to cool.

Add the rest of the ingredients, except the wraps, to the bowl, stirring well as you add each one.

Divide half of the mix between two of the wraps, then roll them in foil and keep cool until ready to eat.

Keep the rest of the chicken and mango filling in the fridge in an airtight container, ready to make up the other two wraps tomorrow.

PER SERVING

KCALS	717
CARBS	97g
PROTEIN	40g
FAT	18g

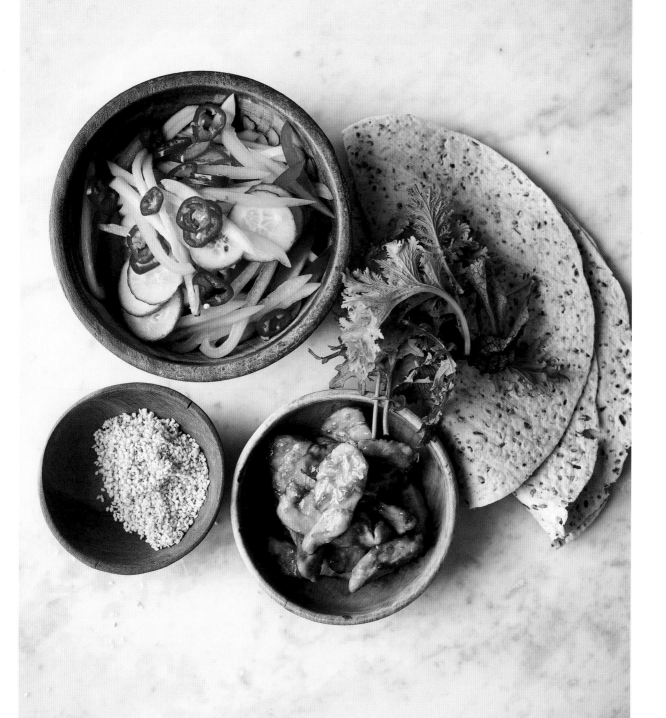

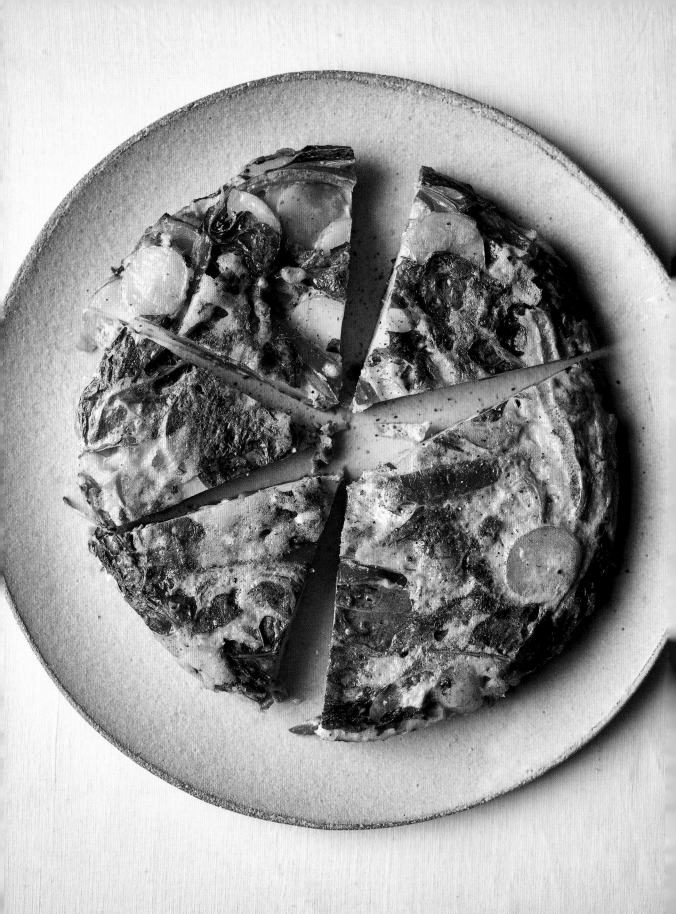

VEGETABLE AND BACON FRITTATA

SERVES 2

2 tbsp olive oil

350g salad potatoes,
   scrubbed and sliced

½ red pepper, sliced

1 garlic clove, crushed

2 smoked bacon rashers,
   chopped

2 tbsp water

3 large eggs

a handful of spinach leaves,
   chopped

salt and pepper

salad and crusty bread,
   to serve

This recipe takes a bit of time to cook but it's well worth the effort and, as it's delicious hot or cold, you can eat one portion hot for supper and then have the other one cold for lunch the next day. It's high in protein and, once you get the hang of it, you can experiment with other ingredients. Vegetarians can drop the bacon and maybe substitute with mushrooms.

Heat the oil in a large non-stick frying pan over a medium heat. Add the potatoes, red pepper, garlic and bacon and sauté for 10 minutes. Make sure you stir and turn everything regularly to avoid them catching.

Add the water to the pan and cook for a further 10 minutes, or until the potatoes are soft.

While the potatoes are cooking, crack the eggs into a large bowl, add a pinch of salt and pepper and whisk well.

Once the potatoes are done, add the contents of the pan to the eggs and mix together, then stir in the chopped spinach, making sure everything is mixed together really well.

Add a little extra oil to the pan, if needed, then pour in the egg and potato mixture. Turn the heat to low and cook for 10–15 minutes, or until the mixture is almost set. Be patient and do not stir it.

Turn the frittata out onto a large dinner plate, slide it back into the pan and cook the other side for a further 2–3 minutes. Alternatively, finish it off under a preheated grill.

Allow to cool, cut into slices and either wrap in foil or put in an airtight container and store in the fridge.

Serve with a salad and some crusty bread.

PER SERVING
(salad and bread
not included)

KCALS	506
CARBS	35g
PROTEIN	20g
FAT	32g

RECOVERY-BOOSTING SMOKED MACKEREL SALAD

SERVES 2

100g quinoa

300ml water

200g (2 fillets) smoked
mackerel, chopped

1 avocado, peeled,
destoned and sliced

2 tomatoes, chopped

1 red pepper, chopped

2 spring onions, sliced

1 tbsp olive oil

1 tsp balsamic vinegar

salt and pepper

This salad is a brilliant option if you want a lighter lunch but don't want to skimp on protein or flavour. Its recovery-boosting qualities are down to the inflammation-moderating properties of the omega-3 fats found in the mackerel and the omega-9 in the avocado. You'll also get a hit of the antioxidant lycopene from the tomatoes and the pepper. This nutrient has been linked to many health benefits including reduced risk of heart disease and cancer.

First, cook the quinoa. Rinse it well under cold water and then place it and the 300ml water in a saucepan over a medium heat.

Bring to the boil then reduce to a simmer and cook until all of the liquid is absorbed. This should take about 10–15 minutes. Set aside and allow to cool completely.

Place the mackerel, avocado and the vegetables in a large bowl with the quinoa, add the olive oil and balsamic vinegar to dress, season with a pinch of salt and pepper and toss thoroughly.

Divide everything between two airtight containers and store in the fridge.

PER SERVING

KCALS	708
CARBS	35g
PROTEIN	31g
FAT	47g

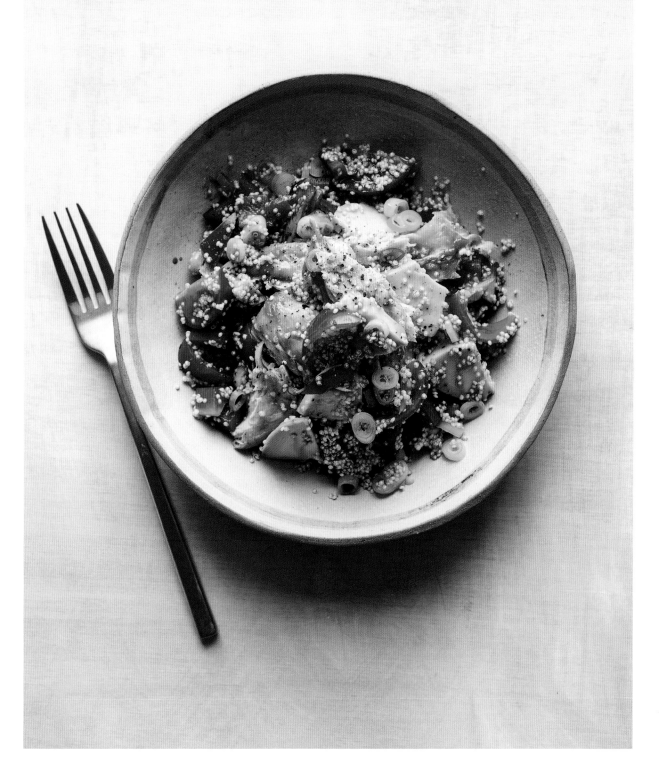

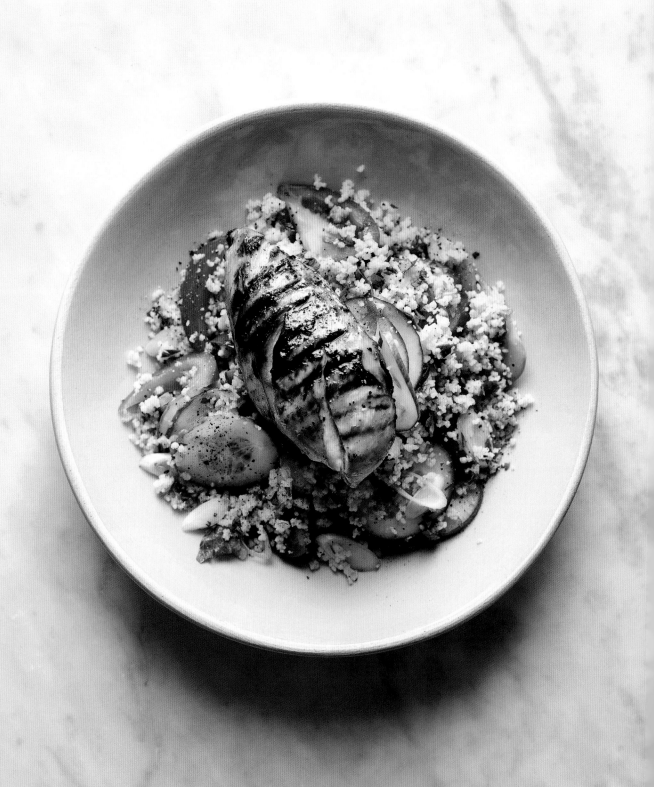

TABBOULEH AND GRILLED SPICY CHICKEN BREASTS

SERVES 2

2 skinless chicken breasts
  (around 200g)

For the marinade

3 tbsp olive oil

1 tsp salt

½ tsp pepper

½ tsp paprika

½ tsp ground cumin

¼ tsp cayenne pepper

2 garlic cloves, crushed

250ml apple juice

For the tabbouleh

125g couscous

250ml water

2 tomatoes, chopped

½ small cucumber, sliced

4 spring onions, sliced

20g parsley, finely chopped

zest and juice of 1 lemon

3 tbsp olive oil

1 garlic clove, crushed

PER SERVING

KCALS	811
CARBS	63g
PROTEIN	43g
FAT	41g

If there's one thing that athletes tend to eat a lot of, it's chicken breasts. Although a great source of lean protein, they can be dry and get a bit monotonous. Marinating them makes a massive difference but most shop-bought marinades are packed with sugar. This homemade one is delicious and only has the apple juice to sweeten it. Tabbouleh is a Middle Eastern salad and, being based around couscous, is a great source of carbs. It's also packed with fresh veg and healthy fats from the olive oil. It's super versatile and is great with any grilled meat or fish.

Make several deep scores across each chicken breast with a sharp knife.

Mix all of the ingredients for the marinade together in a large jug, then pour the marinade into a large ziplock bag. Place the chicken breasts in the bag and put in the fridge to marinate for at least an hour but ideally overnight.

Preheat your grill. Remove the chicken breasts from the marinade and place on a baking tray. Grill until cooked through. Depending on the temperature of your grill and thickness of the chicken breasts this will be 6–8 minutes. If in doubt, cut one open and double check that it is no longer pink.

Set the chicken breasts aside and allow to thoroughly cool.

To make the tabbouleh, put the couscous into a large bowl. Use a kettle to boil the water, pour it over the couscous and cover.

Leave to stand for 5 minutes, or until all the liquid has been absorbed. Separate the couscous grains with a fork and allow to cool.

Add all of the other tabbouleh ingredients to the couscous and mix well.

Divide the couscous between two airtight containers, add a chicken breast to each, and store in the fridge.

GREEK SALAD PITTA BREADS

(VEGETARIAN)

SERVES 2

2 tomatoes, chopped

½ small cucumber, sliced

½ red onion, finely diced

1 garlic clove, finely chopped

½ a 340g jar of sliced
black olives, drained

45g feta cheese, cubed

4 wholemeal pitta breads,
sliced in half

For the dressing

2 tbsp olive oil

½ tsp dried oregano

1 tsp white wine vinegar

salt and pepper

A lighter lunch option that's ideal for days when you might not be training and don't require as many calories. You can also pair it with any grilled meat or fish if you want a more substantial meal. It's a real taste of the sun and, even on a cold winter's day, will remind you of your holidays. With plenty of vegetables, it's high in antioxidants and, because the feta cheese gives you some protein and fat, it'll keep you feeling surprisingly full. Try to use wholemeal pitta breads as these will release their energy slower and keep your blood sugar stable. I'd recommend filling the pitta breads when you're ready to eat, as they can get a bit soggy if made in advance.

Make the dressing in a mug or small jug by whisking the oil, oregano, vinegar and a pinch of salt and pepper together really well using a fork.

Mix all the other ingredients, except the pitta breads, together in a large bowl, pour over the dressing and toss well. Divide between two airtight containers and store in the fridge.

Wrap the pitta breads in foil to keep them fresh and fill them with the Greek salad just before eating.

PER SERVING

KCALS	680
CARBS	68g
PROTEIN	18g
FAT	36g

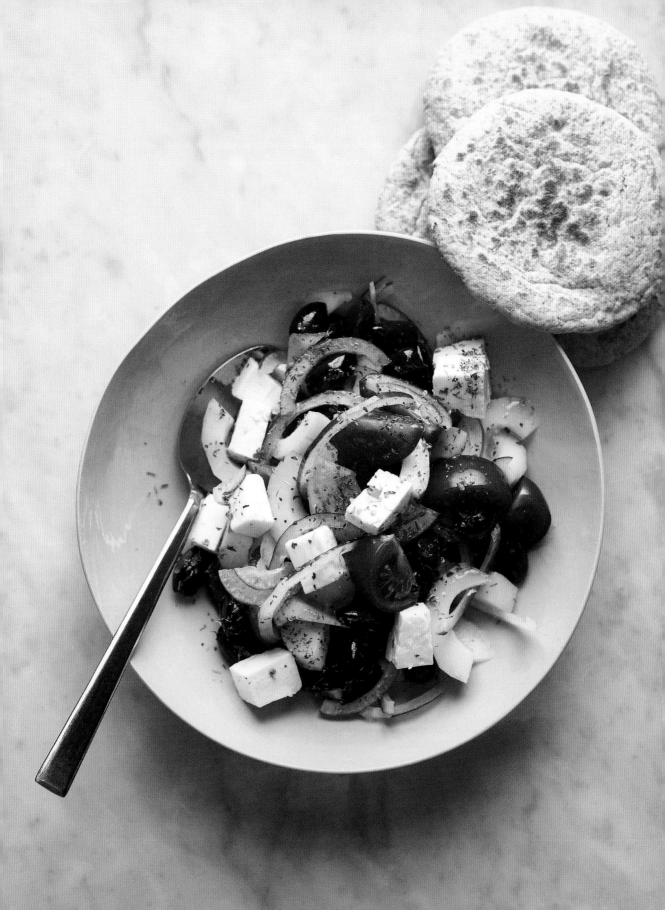

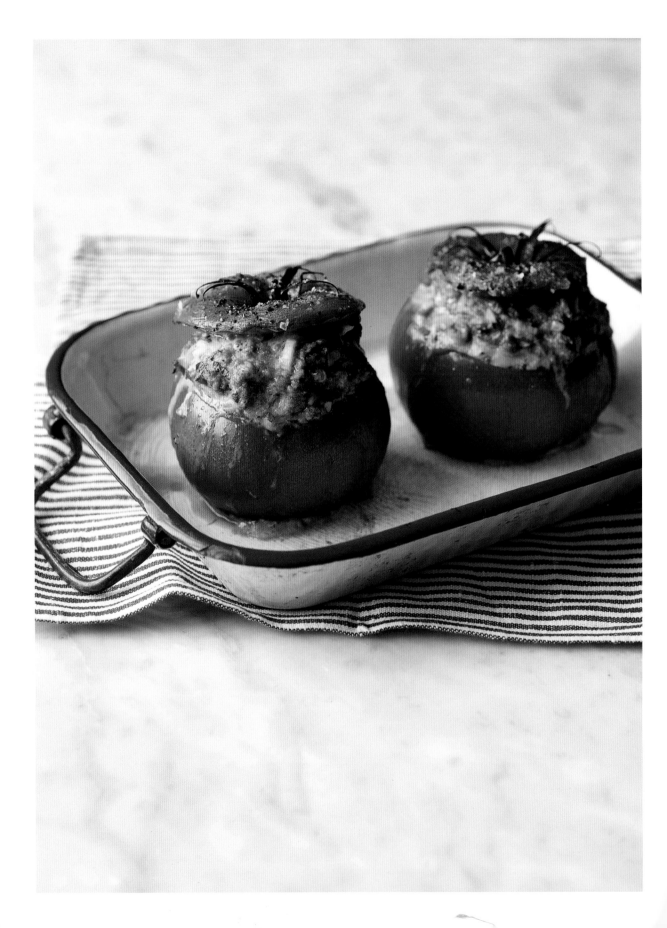

TURKEY-STUFFED BEEF TOMATOES

SERVES 2

2 large beef tomatoes

250g lean turkey mince

1 small onion, finely chopped

1 garlic clove, crushed

1 small egg

2 tsp chopped parsley

½ tsp dried chilli flakes (optional)

salt and pepper

Turkey is an excellent source of high-quality lean protein and this recipe, which uses the tomatoes to hold what's effectively a turkey burger, is brilliant as a portable lunch. For a lower carb day, if you aren't exercising, they're a filling enough lunch on their own but are also great accompanied with salads and/or crusty bread.

Preheat the oven to 180°C/gas mark 4.

Cut a thin slice off the bottom of the tomatoes to give them a flat base and then slice off the top quarter for the lid. Use a spoon to hollow out the tomatoes but leave a decent layer of flesh.

In a bowl, use your hands to thoroughly mix the turkey mince, onion, garlic, egg, parsley and seasoning. I like a bit of spice, so I'd chuck in some chilli flakes, but these are optional.

Stuff the tomatoes with the turkey mince mix, dividing it evenly between the two tomatoes, then put the lids back on. Place on a baking tray and bake in the oven for 30–35 minutes.

Allow to cool, divide between two airtight containers and store in the fridge.

These are great served with some salad greens and my tabbouleh (see page 219) or some crusty bread.

PER SERVING
(salad and bread not included)

KCALS	242
CARBS	11g
PROTEIN	35g
FAT	6g

AVOCADO, TOMATO AND LIME PASTA SALAD
(VEGAN)

SERVES 2

115g wholewheat penne pasta

zest and juice of 1 lime

1 avocado, peeled, destoned and chopped

2 tomatoes, chopped

a handful of fresh coriander, chopped

1 red onion, chopped

1 red chilli, deseeded and finely chopped

A really tasty light lunch that can be eaten on its own or, if you want to add some protein, with some grilled meat or fish. It's packed with vitamins and antioxidants and the avocado gives you plenty of healthy fats. I love the Mexican and Thai flavours in this salad but, if you're not so keen on the heat, you can miss out the chilli.

Cook the pasta according to the packet instructions. It normally takes about 10–12 minutes. Use plenty of vigorously boiling water, and a bit of olive oil can help to stop it sticking together. Once cooked, drain well, put to one side and allow to cool.

Put all of the other ingredients into a bowl, add the pasta and toss thoroughly.

Divide between two airtight containers and store in the fridge.

PER SERVING

KCALS	281
CARBS	33g
PROTEIN	7g
FAT	16g

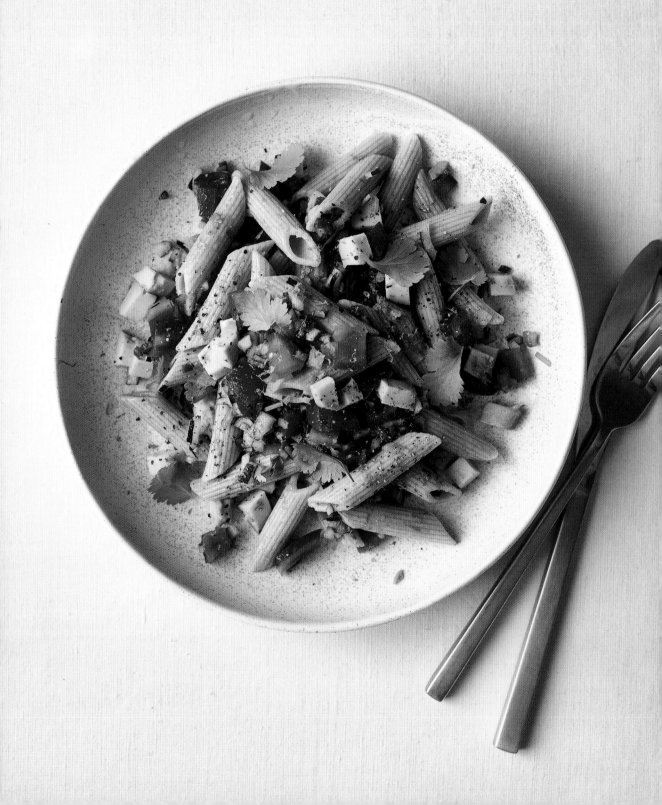

JUST BECAUSE SOMETHING IS HEALTHIER . . .

. . . it doesn't mean you can eat unlimited amounts. This might sound really obvious but it's a common mistake that people make and then wonder why, despite making healthy food choices, they're not making the weight-loss progress they expect or want. Nuts and seeds are a great example of this. They're a brilliant snack choice because they are packed with beneficial fats, such as omega-3, and deliver a decent plant-based protein punch. However, because they're so nutrient dense, if you have a big bowl of mixed nuts and seeds on your desk and mindlessly pick at it all day, it's likely you'll consume an alarming number of calories.

Dried fruit is another good example. Would you eat five fresh apricots in one sitting? Probably not but, with dried fruit, you can do this without even thinking about it. The solution is to divide your snacks into single, measured servings. For nuts, seeds and dried fruit, 30g in total is about right for a snack-sized portion.

Finally, be wary of smoothies as, although they can be super convenient and can deliver a load of great nutrients, they can also be incredibly calorie dense. My Chocolate Protein Thick Shake (page 259) should probably be an occasional treat and definitely not a daily snack option!

DINNERS

Sometimes (usually at the weekend) you might have a bit of time to cook dinner but, more often than not, it's usually a bit of a rush. With this in mind, I've done a mix of quick and slower recipes. All of them serve four so they are perfect for a family and, although healthy, you'd be happy serving them to friends who've come over for dinner. I'm a self-confessed junk-food fan so it's no surprise that there are healthy versions of a burger, pizza and fish and chips here. Apart from the fish and chips, all of these recipes are delicious cold so if you're not feeding four, you've got tomorrow's lunch sorted. The Mixed Bean Chilli and my Rio 2016 Feijoada are also good for freezing. I've created two dinners that are inspired by the two Olympics I've been to and another for the one that's hopefully coming next.

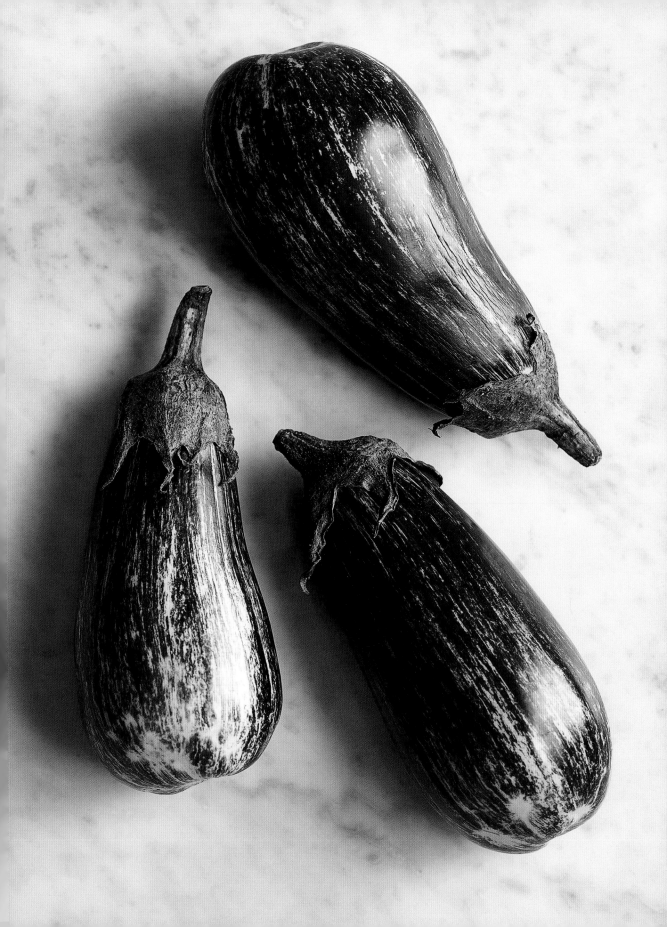

THAI-STYLE TURKEY BURGERS

SERVES 4

2 tsp coconut oil

4 spring onions, chopped

1 tsp grated fresh ginger

1 garlic clove, crushed

1 red chilli, deseeded
and chopped

500g lean turkey mince

20g oats

1 medium egg

zest and juice of ½ lime

a handful of fresh coriander
leaves, roughly torn

I love a burger and these super-healthy but really tasty Thai-style ones are up there with my favourites. Turkey mince is a great source of lean protein that'll help to support muscle growth and recovery post training. You can tailor what you serve the burgers with depending on your activity level that day. If you've taken it easy, just go for a mixed salad, but if you've trained hard, you can go full fast-food fix with buns and my healthy chips (see page 238).

In a frying pan, melt 1 teaspoon of the coconut oil over a medium-low heat. Add the spring onions, ginger, garlic and chilli and sauté for about 5 minutes, stirring occasionally. Take care not to allow the ingredients to burn.

Remove the pan from the heat and, using a slotted spoon, transfer the contents to a large mixing bowl and allow to cool completely.

Once cool, add the turkey mince, oats, egg, lime zest and juice and coriander leaves, then mix everything together thoroughly using your hands.

Divide the mixture into four even-sized patties, transfer to a plate and cover. Place them in the fridge to firm up for 20 minutes–1 hour.

Preheat the oven to 180°C/gas mark 4.

Add the remaining 1 teaspoon of oil to a baking tray, place the tray in the oven for a few minutes to allow the oil to heat up and melt. Carefully transfer the patties to the baking tray and cook for 25–30 minutes, turning halfway through.

Serve with a mixed salad or whatever you fancy.

PER SERVING
(salad not included)

KCALS	215
CARBS	4g
PROTEIN	33g
FAT	7g

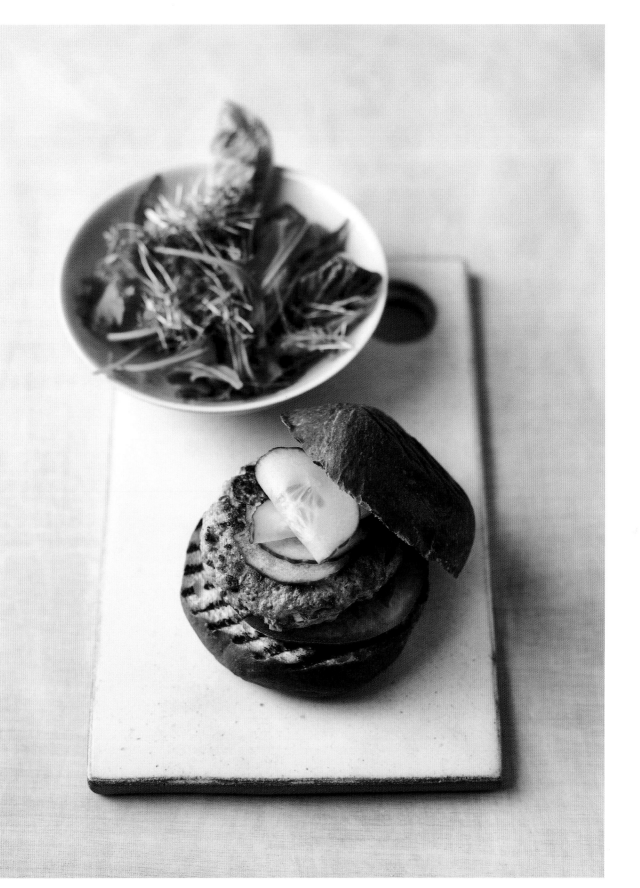

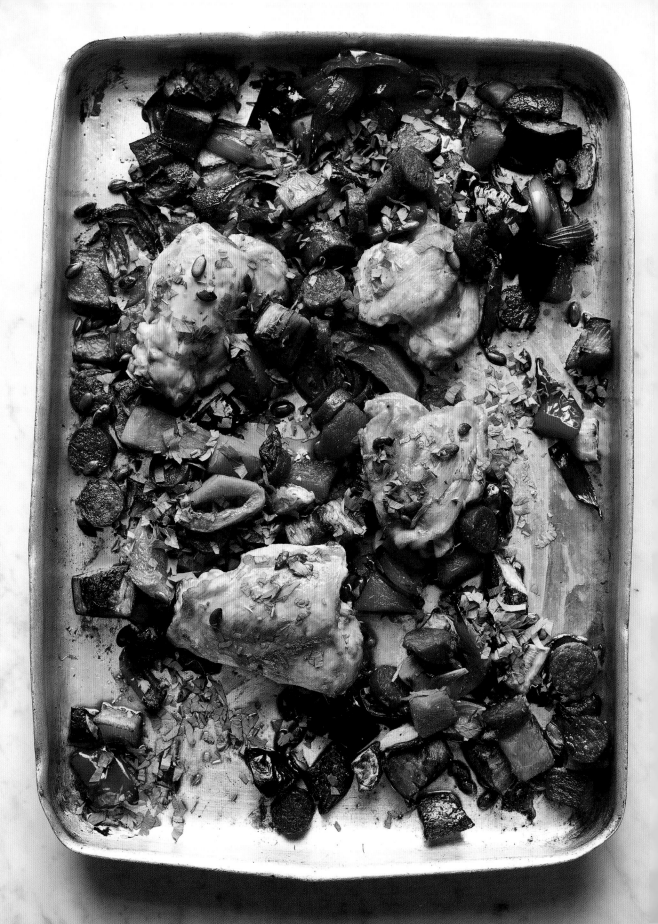

SPANISH-STYLE ROASTED VEG AND CHICKEN TRAY BAKE

SERVES 4

1 tbsp olive oil

1 red onion, chopped

2 garlic cloves, chopped

1 red pepper, chopped

1 butternut squash, peeled and chopped

1 courgette, chopped

1 aubergine, chopped

1 tbsp pumpkin seeds

1 ring of chorizo, skin removed and chopped

4 large skinless chicken breasts

a handful of fresh parsley, chopped

salt and pepper

I love tray bakes like this, mainly because they're so easy and require minimal washing up! This one is delicious. Although the chorizo is a little fatty, a little goes a long way and it gives the dish an amazing deep flavour. The chicken guarantees your protein intake and you get plenty of slow-release carbs from all the vegetables. The pumpkin seeds bring a delicious nutty taste, some crunchy texture and healthy omega-3 fats. It's a complete meal on its own but you might want some crusty bread to mop your plate.

Preheat the oven to 200°C/gas mark 6.

Drizzle the oil into a large roasting tin and place the tin in the oven for a few minutes so the oil heats up.

Remove the roasting tin from the oven and add the onion, garlic, pepper, butternut squash, courgette, aubergine and pumpkin seeds. Mix everything together, ensuring all the ingredients are well covered with oil. Return to the oven for 20 minutes.

Meanwhile, heat a frying pan over a medium heat and add the chorizo. Cook for 5–7 minutes until it has released plenty of its oil. Use a slotted spoon to remove the chorizo, leaving as much of the oil as possible in the pan, and put the chorizo to one side. Carefully place the chicken breasts in the pan. Season with a pinch of salt and pepper and cook for 10 minutes, turning halfway through.

Once the vegetables have been in the oven for 20 minutes, remove the tray and add the chorizo. Mix everything together well, place the chicken breasts on top, and return to the oven for another 20 minutes.

Remove from the oven and stir the fresh parsley through before serving.

PER SERVING
(bread not included)

KCALS	590
CARBS	25g
PROTEIN	52g
FAT	32g

HEALTHY PIZZA
(VEGETARIAN)

SERVES 4
(MAKES 2 PIZZAS)

For the base

200g strong white four

200g strong wholemeal flour

1 tsp easy-blend dried yeast

a pinch of salt

250ml warm water

For the topping

1 tbsp olive oil

1 small onion, finely chopped

1 garlic clove, crushed

1 x 400g tin of chopped
   tomatoes, drained

½ tsp dried basil

½ tsp dried oregano

½ tsp dried parsley

2 handfuls of cherry tomatoes,
   halved

50g mozzarella cheese, sliced

a handful of fresh basil,
   roughly chopped, optional

salt and pepper

PER SERVING

KCALS	451
CARBS	72g
PROTEIN	18g
FAT	8g

Everyone loves a pizza but the problem with many shop-bought and takeaway ones is they often have overly stodgy and doughy bases and far too much cheese and other unhealthy toppings. There's something really satisfying about making your own pizza and you're completely in control of what goes into it – and on top of it. This simple margherita is delicious in its own right but feel free to add whatever extra toppings you fancy. If I'm wanting a bit of extra protein, an egg cracked into the middle is delicious.

First make the topping. Heat half the olive oil in a frying pan over a medium heat and add the onion and garlic. Sauté for 5–7 minutes, or until the onion starts to soften. Reduce the heat, add the tinned tomatoes and dried herbs and cook gently for a further 5 minutes. Remove from the heat and allow to cool.

In a food processor with a dough blade, mix the flours, yeast and salt. Pour in the water and mix into a soft dough. This will take about 5 minutes.

Remove the dough from the food processor, divide into two balls and, on a lightly floured surface, roll out into two bases. Each should be roughly 30cm across or you could make them into ovals. Transfer them carefully onto lightly oiled baking trays.

Spread the tomato sauce evenly onto the bases and then scatter over the cherry tomato halves, mozzarella and any other toppings you fancy. Season with a pinch of salt and pepper. Drizzle with the rest of the olive oil and leave to rise for about 20 minutes.

Meanwhile, preheat the oven to 220°C/gas mark 7.

Bake the pizzas in the oven for 10–12 minutes and scatter with the fresh basil, if wanted, before serving.

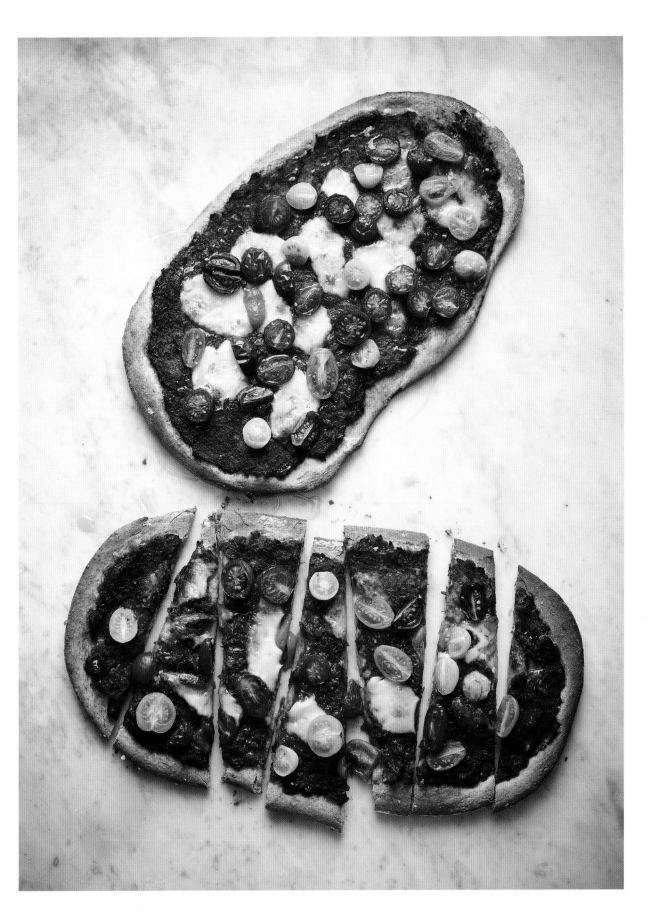

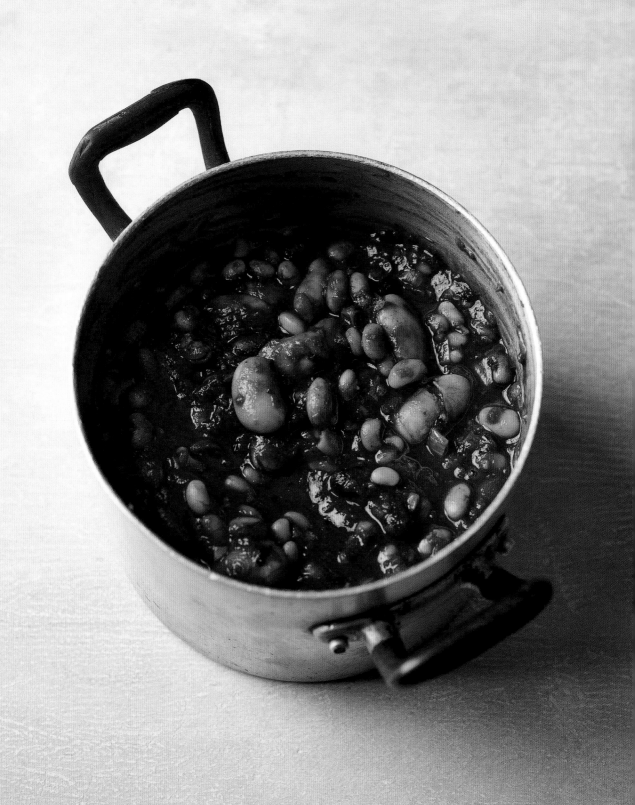

MIXED BEAN CHILLI

(VEGAN)

SERVES 4

100g dried black-eyed peas

100g dried butter beans

100g dried haricot beans

100g dried red kidney beans

100g dried pinto beans

1 tbsp olive oil

2 onions, chopped

1 garlic clove, minced

2 tsp ground cumin

2 tsp ground paprika

2 tsp chilli powder

500ml water

1 vegetable stock cube

1 x 400g tin of chopped tomatoes

1 tbsp tomato purée

50g dark chocolate (preferably
  85% cocoa solids), chopped

a handful of fresh coriander,
  chopped

salt and pepper

rice, to serve

If you're vegan, vegetarian or just trying to cut down on your meat intake, this is a really satisfying and filling option. When served with rice, all of the essential amino acids are represented and so it's an excellent source of protein. It's also a great choice for batch cooking and freezing some portions so you always have a healthy meal ready to go. The beans will need to be soaked overnight in cold water, so it requires a bit of planning. The chocolate might seem like a weird ingredient but, trust me, it adds real depth of flavour. Just make sure you use one with a high cocoa content, ideally 85%.

Rinse all the beans well under cold water, place in a large bowl, cover with water and leave to soak overnight. Drain well.

In a large saucepan, heat the olive oil over a medium heat. Add the onions and garlic and sauté for 5–7 minutes, or until the onions start to soften. Add the cumin, paprika, chilli powder and a splash of water, then lower the heat and cook for a further 5 minutes.

Boil the 500ml of water in a kettle, pour it into a jug, and dissolve the stock cube in it.

Add the tinned tomatoes, tomato purée and stock to the saucepan, turn the heat back up and bring to a simmer. Add the beans and chocolate, and a pinch of salt and pepper. Stir well, pop the lid on and turn the heat back down to low.

Cook for 40 minutes–1 hour, stirring occasionally, until the liquid has been reduced and the beans are soft.

Stir through the chopped coriander and serve with rice.

PER SERVING
(rice not included)

KCALS	548
CARBS	81g
PROTEIN	31g
FAT	12g

LONDON 2012 HEALTHY FISH AND CHIPS

SERVES 4

For the chips

1kg floury potatoes, such as Maris Piper, peeled and sliced into chips

1 tsp olive oil

salt and pepper

For the fish

1 slice of white bread

50g oats

2 medium eggs

4 white fish fillets (120g each), such as cod or haddock

2 tbsp plain white flour

salt and pepper

To serve

mushy peas

salt and vinegar

PER SERVING
(mushy peas
not included)

KCALS	425
CARBS	58g
PROTEIN	32g
FAT	6g

Here is the first of my Olympic-inspired dinners – and what says Britain more than fish and chips! Unfortunately, despite being undeniably delicious, the real thing is not really a healthy choice. However, my oven-baked version slashes the calories and saturated fat but still tastes great. White fish is an excellent lean protein source, and you can serve the healthy chips with loads of other things.

Place two large baking trays inside the oven and preheat it to 200°C/gas mark 6.

Bring some water to the boil in a large saucepan, add the chips and cook for 4 minutes. Drain well.

Remove one of the baking trays from the oven, tip the chips onto it, drizzle over the olive oil, season and then turn with a spatula to ensure all the chips are coated with oil. Place in the oven and bake for 15 minutes.

While the chips are in the oven, start making the fish. Toast the slice of bread and then blitz it in a food processor with the oats and a pinch of salt and pepper. Spread the mix out evenly onto a large plate.

Beat the eggs in a large bowl.

Lightly dust each fish fillet with the flour, shake off the excess and dip them in the egg, then roll them in the breadcrumbs to cover.

When the chips have been in the oven for the 15 minutes, take them out and turn them. Take out the second baking tray and place the fish fillets on it. Put both trays back in the oven for 20 minutes. Turn the fish halfway through.

Remove the fish and chips from the oven and serve with peas and plenty of salt and vinegar.

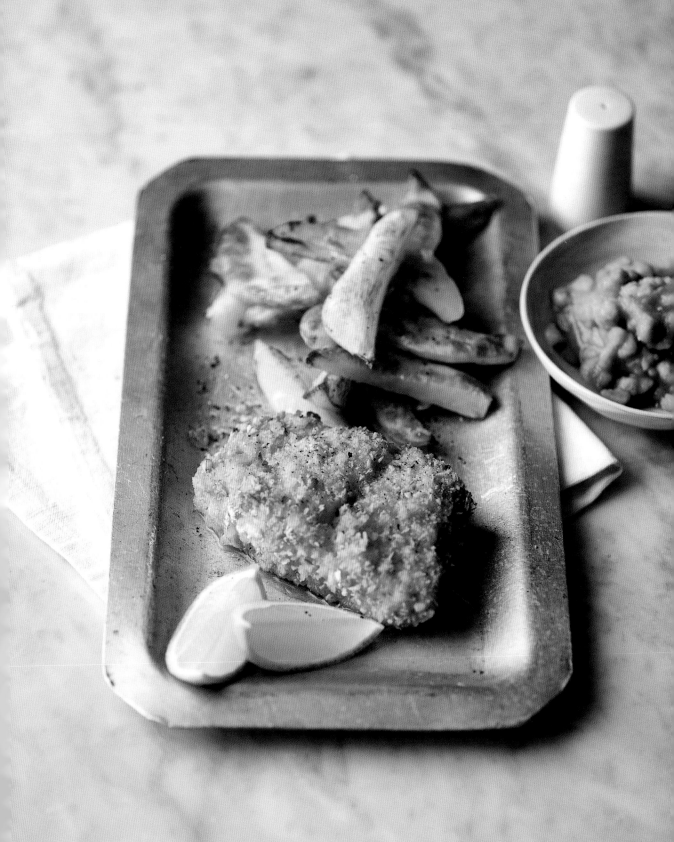

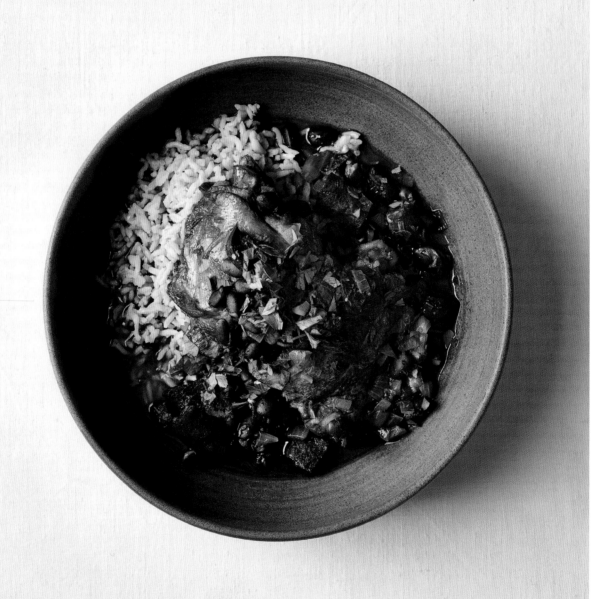

RIO 2016 FEIJOADA

SERVES 4

250g dried black beans

1 ring of chorizo, skin removed and chopped

8 skinless bone-in chicken thighs

100g streaky smoked bacon, sliced

1 tsp olive oil

2 large onions, chopped

4 garlic cloves, crushed

a pinch of chilli flakes

2 bay leaves

2 tbsp white wine vinegar

a handful of fresh parsley, chopped

salt and pepper

rice, to serve

This hearty traditional Brazilian stew wasn't on my pre-competition menu but, once I had the gold medal in the bag, I was able to enjoy it a few times. The real version uses pork rib and pork shoulder but, for a leaner, faster alternative, I use chicken thighs. It's packed with flavour and protein, and with a generous serving of rice, really hits the comfort spot on a cold winter's day.

Rinse the beans well under cold water, place in a large bowl, cover with water and leave to soak overnight. Drain well.

Place a large heavy-based saucepan over a medium heat. Add the chorizo and cook for 5–7 minutes until it has released plenty of its oil, then remove from the pan with a slotted spoon, leaving as much of the oil behind as possible. Set aside the chorizo.

Put the chicken thighs into the chorizo oil in the pan and seal for 5 minutes on each side. Remove the chicken and set aside.

Add the bacon to the pan and cook for 5 minutes, or until crispy. Remove and set aside with the chicken and the chorizo.

Add the olive oil to the pan, followed by the onion, garlic and chilli flakes. Sauté for 5–7 minutes, or until the onions start to soften.

Return the meat to the pan along with the beans, bay leaves, vinegar and a pinch of salt and pepper. Add enough water to cover, bring to the boil and then put the lid on, reduce to a simmer and cook for 1 hour or until most of the liquid has been absorbed and the beans are soft.

Sprinkle over the fresh parsley and serve with rice.

PER SERVING
(rice not included)

KCALS	867
CARBS	21g
PROTEIN	71g
FAT	48g

TOKYO 2020 TURKEY TERIYAKI STIR-FRY

SERVES 4

500g turkey breast,
  cut into strips

1 tbsp peanut oil

1 red onion, chopped

1 green pepper, finely sliced

½ red chilli, deseeded
  and finely sliced

rice or noodles, to serve

For the marinade/sauce

60ml dark soy sauce

1 tbsp runny honey

1 tbsp white wine vinegar

1 tbsp sesame oil

1 tbsp dark brown sugar

1 tbsp sesame seeds

1 garlic clove, crushed

1 tsp finely chopped
  fresh ginger

2 tbsp water

I don't want to count my chickens, but hopefully in 2020 I'll be at my third Olympics and will get the chance to sample Japanese culture and food in Tokyo. Until then, I'll make do with my teriyaki-style stir-fry. It's really simple to make and, as long as you're organised enough to marinate the turkey the night before, it's probably one of the quickest meals you can cook.

Put all of the marinade ingredients into a large bowl and whisk together really well.

Add the turkey breast strips to the marinade, cover, place in the fridge and marinate for at least an hour but ideally overnight.

Heat the oil in a non-stick wok over a high heat. Using a slotted spoon, remove the turkey from the marinade and stir-fry for 3 minutes. Add the onions, pepper and chilli and stir-fry for another 3 minutes, then pour the marinade into the wok and stir-fry for a final 1–2 minutes.

Serve with rice or noodles.

PER SERVING
(rice or noodles
not included)

KCALS	266
CARBS	14g
PROTEIN	30g
FAT	10g

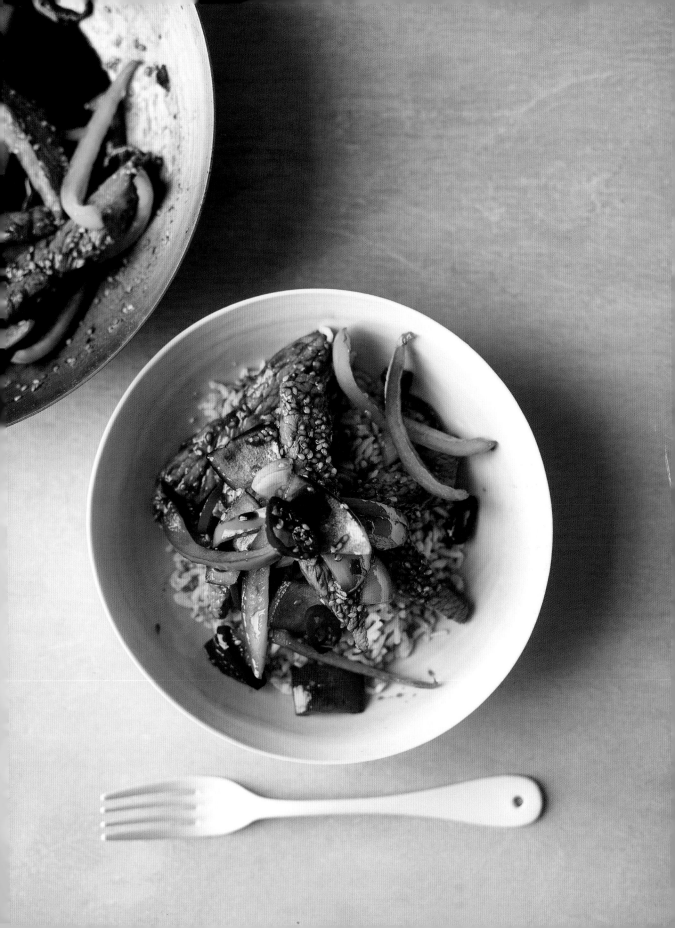

SNACK BEFORE BEDTIME?

It's thought that your body recovers from exercise, repairs itself and makes the physiological adaptations that result in you getting fitter when you're asleep. I know personally how important sleep is to me and my performance in competition and training, and that if I'm not getting a quality 10–11 hours a night, my performance begins to decline. So, if your body is doing all this work for you while you're sleeping, should you be giving it a bit of fuel before you go to bed? If you're eating an overly restrictive or inadequate diet, you may wake up during the night feeling ravenously hungry and probably raid the fridge. However, even if you are eating well, a small snack before bedtime, especially if you've trained that day, can help with sleep and adaptation.

This shouldn't be anything substantial; a small serving of yoghurt (175g) is perfect. Yoghurt contains the amino acid tryptophan which helps to produce the feel-good chemical serotonin and the relaxing and sleep-inducing chemical melatonin. It's also packed with beneficial bacteria which will help to populate your gut and aid digestion. The milk proteins help with muscle development and preservation. Finally, it'll stave off midnight sugar cravings.

SNACKS
AND TREATS

Regular snacking or grazing is important for keeping your blood sugar stable throughout the day and ensuring that you have enough energy and focus for training, work or whatever else you may be doing. If you don't snack, especially mid-morning, mid-afternoon and pre/post workout, your performance may drop, which can manifest in your inability to finish a workout, poor concentration for an important spreadsheet or getting irritable with your kids. If you've just trained, you'll compromise your recovery if you don't have at least a small snack afterwards, and therefore the gains from the workout you've just done and your performance in your next. It'll make you feel overly hungry at your next main meal, which can mean you're more likely to overeat. Finally, if someone does crack out a packet of biscuits, if you're ravenously hungry and haven't got anything healthier to hand, will you stop at just one?

I'll always ensure that I have some healthy snacks to hand – whether at home, in my kit bag or stashed away somewhere handy if I'm out and about with Leah and Willow. A lot of the time, it'll just be something simple, such as an apple, pear or banana, or a serving of mixed nuts and seeds, but I also like to mix things up and to feel as though I'm having a bit of a treat.

These snacks are all super simple to make and, apart from the ice lollies and the smoothies, are brilliant to take with you on the go.

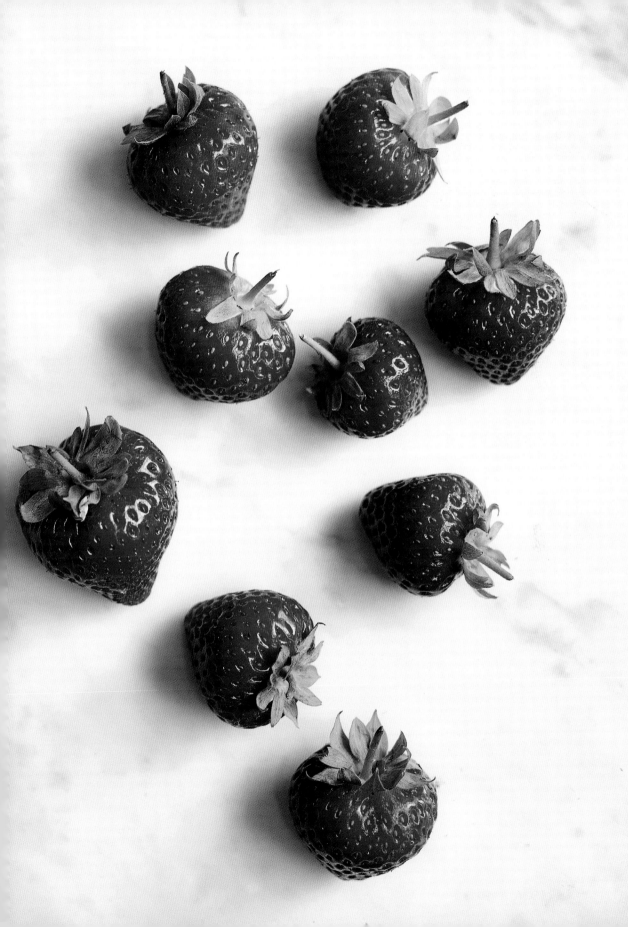

NUT BUTTER-STUFFED DATES (VEGAN)

MAKES 6–9 STUFFED DATES (A SERVING IS 2–3 DATES)

MAKES 24 SERVINGS OF NUT BUTTER (1 SERVING = 1 TBSP)

150g raw almonds

150g raw pistachio kernels

150g raw pecans

½ tsp salt

6–9 Medjool dates
(try to get fat, juicy ones)

These are a super-easy snack, especially if you use shop-bought nut butter! However, it's also really simple to make your own nut butter, and if you do then you can customise it to your tastes. The dates give you a quick energy boost and satisfy any sugar cravings you might have. The nut butter is packed with protein and healthy fats and, because of this, these little mouthfuls are really filling and satisfying. When making the nut butter, you can experiment with different flavours and textures – try cacao, various seeds, vanilla extract, or whatever you fancy.

Preheat your oven to 180°C/gas mark 4.

Spread all the nuts out on a shallow baking tray and pop them in the oven. Roast for 8–12 minutes, until they're golden brown and starting to smell deliciously nutty. Be careful not to burn them.

Put the roasted nuts, still warm, into a food processor and blend until a creamy nut butter forms. Have faith and be patient. They'll first take on a flour-like texture, then they'll start to clump, but they will finally turn into a butter. This can take 10–12 minutes and you might need to scrape the mix back down into the bowl.

Once it's creamy, add the salt. At this stage you can also experiment with some other flavourings and ingredients, if you want.

Transfer the nut butter into clean jars or containers. It'll keep in the fridge for 3 weeks.

To stuff the dates, slice each in half lengthways, remove the stone, fill the space with nut butter and push the halves back together. Then pop them in the fridge for an hour or so to firm up.

You'll have loads of nut butter left over but it's a super-versatile, tasty and healthy snack to have in your fridge.

COMBINED
(1 SERVING
NUT BUTTER
+ 3 DATES)

KCALS	314
CARBS	58g
PROTEIN	4g
FAT	11g

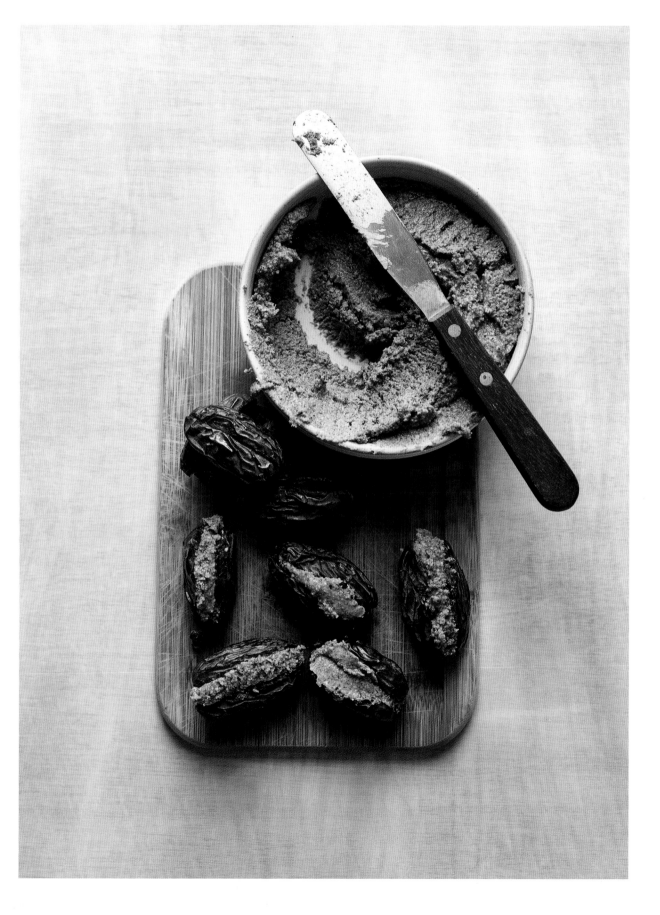

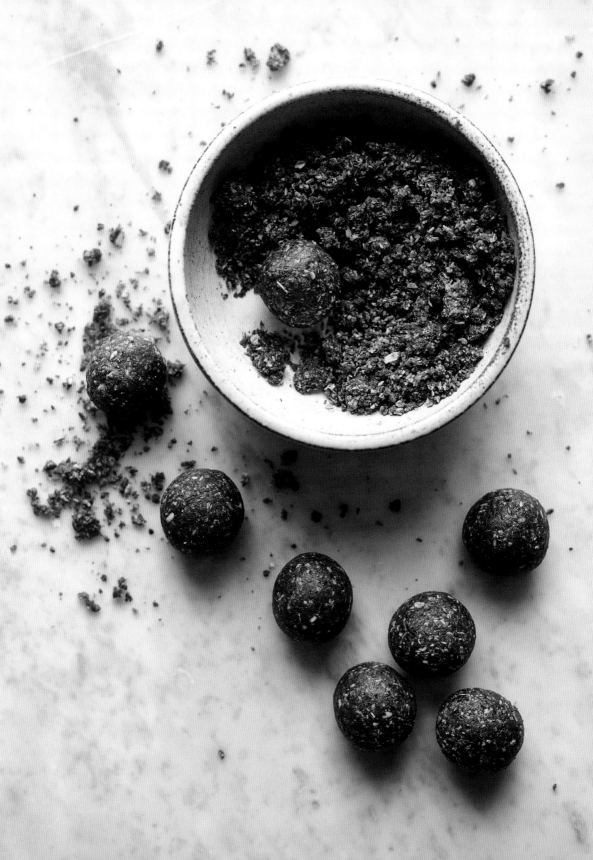

PROTEIN ENERGY BALLS

(VEGAN)

MAKES 10–12 BALLS

A SERVING IS 1–2 BALLS

90g rolled oats

125g almond butter (bought
  or homemade, see page 248)

35g ground flaxseeds

2 tbsp mixed dried fruit

3 dates, pitted

1 tbsp maple syrup

1 tsp cinnamon

These are an amazingly filling snack and are perfect for when you're on the go. The oats give you slow-release carbs for sustained energy, the dried fruit and syrup provide an instant energy boost and the nut butter a decent protein and healthy fat hit. The flaxseeds are high in omega-3, which can help to manage inflammation after a tough workout. You can also experiment with different ingredients. Try swapping the flaxseeds for cacao if you want a chocolatey option, roll the balls in desiccated coconut or add some chopped nuts.

Simply put all the ingredients into a food processor and blitz until well mixed. You'll know they're blended enough when the mixture starts to ball a bit in the blender and it's no longer too tacky to handle.

Roll into balls with your hands; they should be about the circumference of a 2p coin.

If you can resist tucking in straight away, place them in the fridge to set for about 20 minutes.

They'll keep for about a week in a sealed container in the fridge, or they freeze really well and are good for 3 months.

PER PROTEIN BALL

KCALS	141
CARBS	12g
PROTEIN	4g
FAT	8g

STRAWBERRY AND BANANA ICE LOLLIES

(VEGAN)

MAKES 6–8 LOLLIES

1 x 400ml tin of coconut milk

300g strawberries
(fresh or frozen)

1 banana, sliced

3 tbsp agave nectar

Who doesn't love an ice lolly on a hot day, especially if you've just done a tough workout? Unfortunately, a lot of ready-made lollies are packed with sugar and artificial ingredients. My versions are really tasty and the coconut milk not only gives them a lovely creamy texture but also provides a number of health benefits, such as providing medium-chain triglycerides (MCTs), which have been linked to weight loss. You'll need lolly moulds, but these are cheap to buy. You can substitute the strawberries with any berries you like.

Place all the ingredients in a blender and blend until the mixture is smooth. At this stage you'll have a delicious smoothie, but try to resist the temptation to down it!

Pour the mixture into the lolly moulds. Fill them almost to the brim but allow a bit of a gap as the mixture will expand as it freezes.

Freeze for at least 4 hours.

Enjoy in the sun!

PER SERVING

KCALS	189
CARBS	17g
PROTEIN	1g
FAT	12g

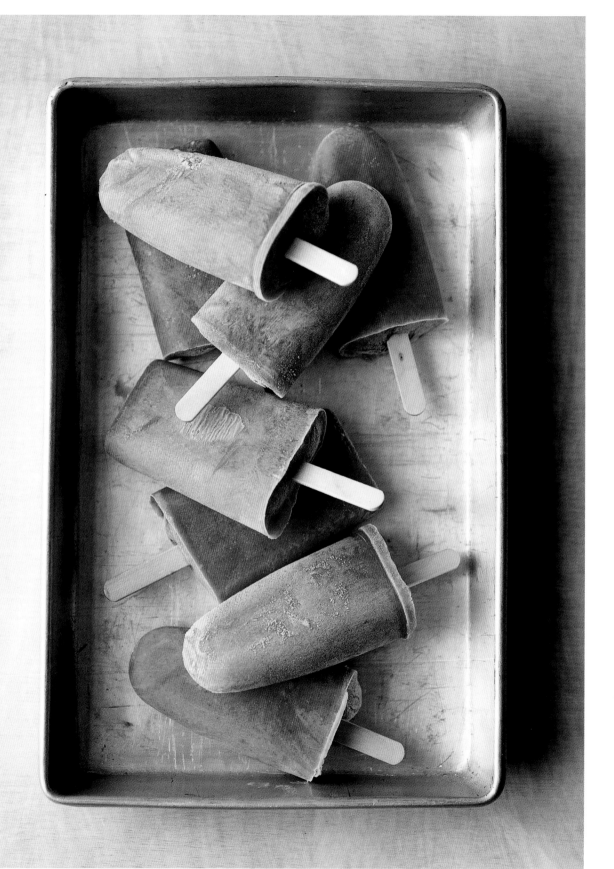

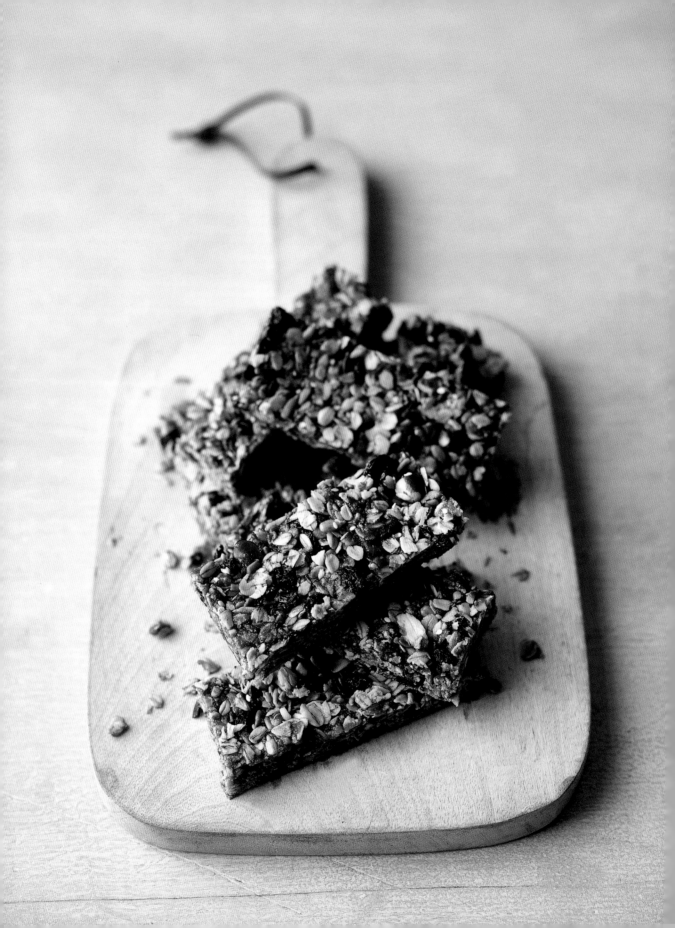

HEALTHY FLAPJACKS
(VEGAN)

MAKES 10 FLAPJACKS

100g coconut oil

140g brown sugar

30g agave nectar

170g oats

75g mixed nuts and seeds,
   chopped

75g mixed dried fruit, chopped

Although these flapjacks are undoubtably healthier than traditional butter and golden syrup ones, they're still fairly high in sugar and are also calorie dense, so you don't want to be eating them daily. However, they're great as a treat, a source of energy for a bike ride or a hike, or if you just want to make yourself popular in the office. You get rapidly available energy from the sugar, agave nectar and dried fruit and then slower-release energy from the oats, seeds, nuts and coconut oil.

Preheat the oven to 160°C/gas mark 3.

Line a 20cm square cake tin with baking paper.

Melt the coconut oil, sugar and agave together in a pan over a low–medium heat. Be careful that the mixture doesn't burn or that the sugar starts to caramelise.

Remove from the heat and tip in the oats, nuts and seeds, and dried fruit. Mix well, ensuring that all the ingredients are coated. Transfer the mixture to the tin and pack it in using the back of a spoon.

Bake for 30–35 minutes until lightly golden and crisp around the edges. Keep an eye on it as it can burn quite quickly.

Leave to cool in the tin. Once cool, turn it out carefully and slice into 10 squares.

The flapjacks will keep in an airtight container in the fridge for 3 days, but I doubt they'll last that long!

PER SERVING

KCALS	280
CARBS	34g
PROTEIN	4g
FAT	14g

BANANA AND OAT MUFFINS

(VEGAN)

MAKES 12 MUFFINS

olive oil, for greasing

70g coconut oil

150g agave nectar

2 eggs

2 ripe bananas, mashed

60ml soya milk

½ tsp cinnamon

1 tsp vanilla extract

1 tsp baking soda

½ tsp salt

30g oats, plus extra for sprinkling

240g wholemeal flour

These muffins are brilliant as an on-the-go breakfast option, as a snack if you need an energy boost an hour or so before a workout or just as a tasty treat. The oats, flour and bananas give you carbs, and the agave syrup a quick energy boost. You also get some protein from the eggs and soya milk and some healthy fats from the coconut oil.

Preheat the oven to 170°C/gas mark 3 and lightly grease a 12-hole muffin tin with olive oil.

In a bowl, mix together the coconut oil, agave nectar, eggs, bananas and soya milk into a smooth batter. You may need to gently heat or quickly microwave the coconut oil to make it liquid. Add the cinnamon, vanilla extract, baking soda and salt, and mix again. Finally, stir in the oats and the flour and mix everything together really well.

Divide the mixture evenly between the holes of the muffin tin and sprinkle over some extra oats. Bake for about 25 minutes, or until a skewer inserted into the middle of one comes out clean.

Allow to cool before turning them out of the tin.

They're best eaten as soon as possible but, if put into an airtight container, will keep in the fridge for up to a week.

PER SERVING
(1 muffin)

KCALS	219
CARBS	35g
PROTEIN	5g
FAT	8g

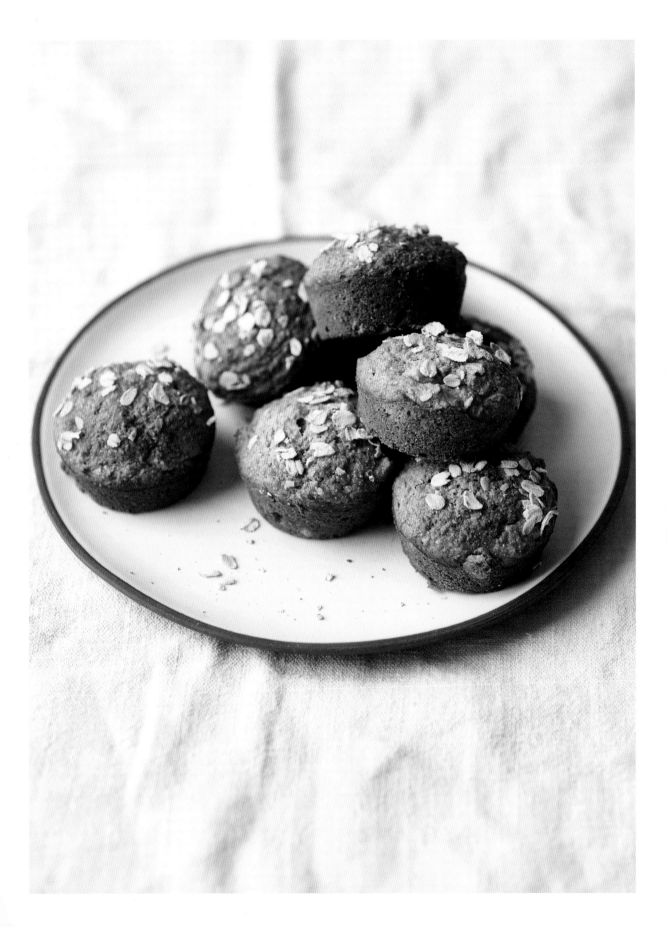

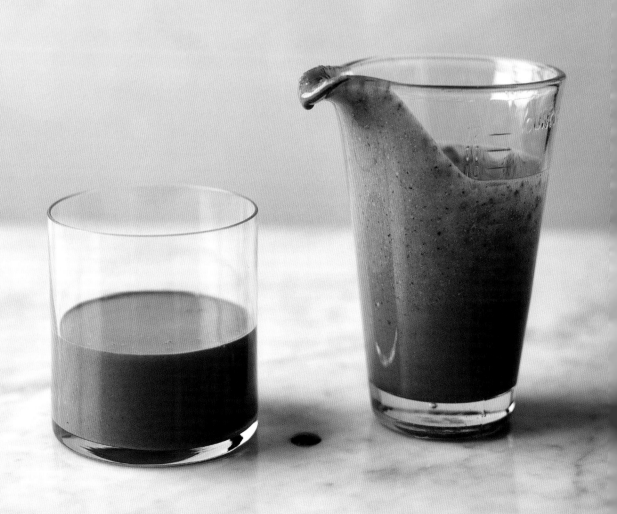

CHOCOLATE PROTEIN THICK SHAKE (VEGAN)

MAKES 1 SMOOTHIE

25g chocolate-flavoured
protein powder (I like My Protein)

200ml unsweetened almond milk

1 generous tbsp nut butter
(bought or homemade,
see page 248)

This is a great protein hit for after a tough workout. It's satisfyingly thick and almost feels like a meal in its own right. For a real fast-food treat at home, you could even have one of these with my turkey burger recipe! You can always vary the flavour depending on what protein powder you use. If you're vegan, there are now some really good-quality, tasty vegan protein powders.

Chuck everything into the blender and give it a thorough blitzing.

Ideally drink this straight away but if you do need to put it in the fridge for later, give it a good shake before drinking as it might have separated slightly.

PER SERVING

KCALS	262
CARBS	4g
PROTEIN	26g
FAT	15g

5-A-DAY+ SUPER SMOOTHIE

(VEGAN)

MAKES 1 SMOOTHIE

80g ripe cantaloupe melon, chopped

80g mixed frozen berries

80g frozen spinach

1 kiwi, peeled and chopped

1 apple, chopped

juice of ½ a lime

1 sprig of fresh mint

250ml water

We're often told to ensure we get our 5 a day but, to stay healthy, 5 portions of fruit and vegetables a day should be the absolute minimum you consume. This super smoothie will deliver your 5 a day and more in one delicious and refreshing nutrient-packed drink. Also, because it doesn't contain extra fruit juice, unnecessary sugar is kept to a minimum.

Chuck everything into the blender and give it a thorough blitzing.

Ideally drink it straight away because it will likely start to discolour, although the lime juice will prevent this to some extent.

PER SERVING

KCALS	170
CARBS	36g
PROTEIN	5g
FAT	2g

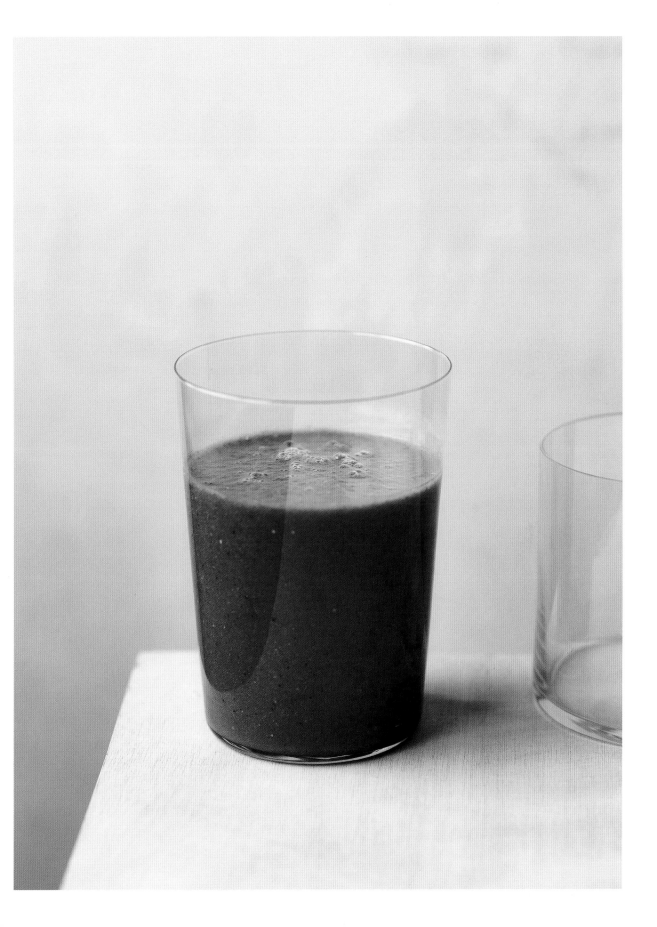

WHEN TO SNACK

Getting the most out of your snacks is largely about timing. If you're eating a healthy and well-timed breakfast, lunch and dinner, my general advice is to try to snack mid-morning and mid-afternoon to avoid blood sugar drops. However, you'll hopefully be doing one of my workouts during the day, so, how best do you fuel those?

If you're working out in the morning, you might be able to perform one of my workouts in a fasted state before breakfast but I wouldn't recommend this if you're fairly new to training or have progressed to the more advanced workouts because you might not have the energy to get through the session. An easily digestible carbohydrate-based snack, such as a banana or a glass of fruit juice, is ideal, and you can get away with having this 10 minutes or so before training. You'd then have your breakfast as usual, which should take care of your recovery nutrients, and then a mid-morning snack.

If you're training at lunchtime, your mid-morning snack should see you through your workout and then you can have lunch afterwards followed by a mid-afternoon snack.

Evening workouts can be a bit trickier to manage depending on when you tend to have your dinner. If you're training before dinner, if it has only been 2–4 hours since your mid-afternoon snack, that should see you through your workout. If it has been longer, go for the pre-workout banana or juice option to give you a bit of a boost. For post-workout, if you'll be eating dinner within an hour or so, there's no need for another snack. However, if it's likely to be longer, a small snack, maybe a Nut Butter-stuffed Date or two or a Protein Energy Ball, will kickstart your recovery and see you through to dinner.

Snacking is really just about supplementing your main meals to ensure you have the energy to perform your workouts and the nutrients to fuel your recovery and adaptation. It's also about maintaining stable blood sugar levels throughout the day. This means that, like your meals, you probably won't snack the same every day. Your snacking should be based on what you're doing and how you're feeling.

INDEX

RECIPE INDEX

First published in 2020 by Headline Home
an imprint of Headline Publishing Group

1

Cataloguing in Publication Data is available from the British Library

Images on pages 6, 15, 16 and 21 © the author
P.9, top © Sport in Pictures/Alamy
P.9, bottom © Andy Hooper/Associated Newspapers/Shutterstock
P.12 © Dmitri Lovetsky/AP/Shutterstock
P.19 © Xinhua News Agency/Shuttershock

Hardback ISBN 978 1 4722 6814 3
eISBN 978 1 4722 6813 6

Yoga mat, step-up box and Olympic rings kindly provided by Jordan Fitness, www.jordanfitness.com

Text with Nikalas Cook
Publishing Director: Lindsey Evans
Senior Editor: Kate Miles
Designed by Nathan Burton
Photography: Dan Jones
Food Styling: Joss Herd
Food Styling Assistant: Hattie Arnold
Prop Styling: Lydia Brun
Nutritionist: Abbie Rudman, BANT-Registered Nutritionist, BSc (Hons) NT, DipBCNH mCNHC.
    (www.thrivenutritionalhealth.com)
Copy Editor: Sophie Elletson
Proofreader: Margaret Gilbey
Indexer: Caroline Wilding

Printed and bound in Italy by L.E.G.O.S.p.A
Colour reproduction by Alta Image

Headline's policy is to use papers that are natural, renewable and recyclable products and
made from wood grown in sustainable forests. The logging and manufacturing processes
are expected to conform to the environmental regulations of the country of origin.

HEADLINE PUBLISHING GROUP
An Hachette UK Company
Carmelite House
50 Victoria Embankment
London EC4Y 0DZ

www.headline.co.uk
www.hachette.co.uk

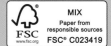

THANKS

Writing this book has been a very exciting experience: putting a lot of what I have learnt over the years into it will hopefully help and inspire many people. It is a very proud moment for me in my career.

I want to thank all the people who have helped make this possible. My family have all been amazing. My wife Leah and my daughter Willow have been a huge driving force with this project and we've all been working out and cooking together at home.

Thank you to everyone at Headline Home, in particular Lindsey Evans, Kate Miles, Sophie Elletson, Rosie Margesson, Viviane Bassett, Tina Paul, Siobhan Hooper and Rob Chilver. Thanks also to the photography and design team: Dan Jones, Heather B and Nathan Burton.

Headline Home and Nikalas Cook have been unbelievably supportive and have helped me curate the book exactly how I envisioned it to be.

I'd like to thank Nick Walters at David Luxton Associates and my agent Hugo Jafari for their invaluable input and feedback.

Finally, I want to add a huge thank you to everyone who has supported me over the years, throughout my career. I love what I do and the support pushes me and motivates me to keep aiming to hit the highest targets.

Many thanks

Max

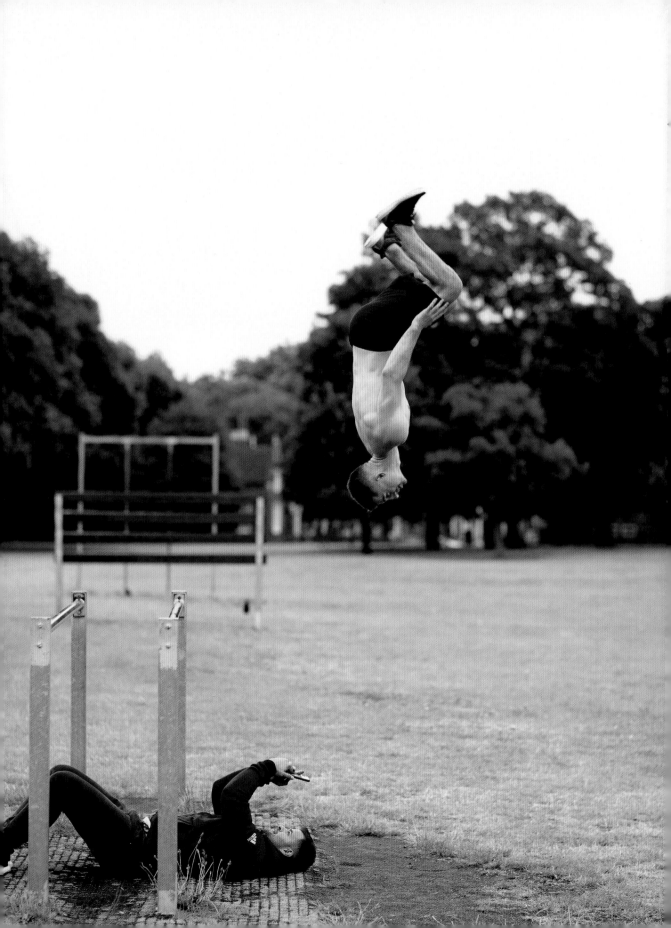